Hand Trembling,

Frenzy Witchcraft,

and Moth Madness

Hand Trembling,

Frenzy Witchcraft,

and Moth Madness

A STUDY OF NAVAJO

SEIZURE DISORDERS

Jerrold E. Levy

Raymond Neutra

Dennis Parker

THE UNIVERSITY OF

ARIZONA PRESS

TUCSON

First paperbound printing 1995

THE UNIVERSITY OF ARIZONA PRESS
Copyright © 1987
The Arizona Board of Regents
All Rights Reserved

This book was set in 10 on 12 Linotron 202 Trump Mediaeval.
Manufactured in the U.S.A.
⊚ This book is printed on acid-free, archival-quality paper.
Designed by Laury A. Egan

Library of Congress Cataloging-in-Publication Data

Levy, Jerrold E., 1930–
    Hand trembling, frenzy witchcraft, and moth madness.

    Bibliography: p.
    Includes index.
    1. Navajo Indians—Medicine.   2. Navajo Indians—
Mental health   3. Psychiatry, Transcultural—Southwest,
New.   4. Convulsions—Cross-cultural studies.
5. Indians of North America—Southwest, New—Medicine.
6. Indians of North America—Southwest, New—Mental
health.   I. Neutra, Raymond. II. Parker, Dennis,
1912–1984.   III. Title.   [DNLM: 1. Attitude to Health.
2. Culture.   3. Epilepsy.   4. Indians, North American—
psychology.   WL 385 L668h]
E99.N3L6   1987   614.5'9853   87-19445
ISBN 0-8165-1036-9 (alk. paper)
ISBN 0-8165-1572-7 (pbk.: alk. paper)

British Cataloguing-in-Publication Data
A catalogue record for this book is available from the British Library.

Contents

Acknowledgments ix

CHAPTER 1 Introduction 1

CHAPTER 2 The Healing Tradition 19

CHAPTER 3 Beliefs About Seizures 39

CHAPTER 4 The Epidemiology of Seizures and Pseudoseizures 60

CHAPTER 5 Navajo Diagnosis and Treatment 87

CHAPTER 6 Hand Trembling 102

CHAPTER 7 Frenzy Witchcraft 119

CHAPTER 8 Moth Madness 133

CHAPTER 9 Ambivalence, Anxiety, and Incest 150

Notes 171

Bibliography 177

Index 189

Tables

4.1   Disposition of Cases   73
4.2   Prevalence Rates in Rochester, Minnesota, and in
      Indian Tribes   74
4.3   Etiology of Epilepsy   74
4.4   Chi-square Analysis of Etiologies   75
4.5   Prevalence of Emotional and Social Problems
      Among Epileptics   80
4.6   Age at Onset of Problems   81
4.7   Clinical Description of Individuals With
      Psychological and Emotional Problems   82–84
4.8   Severity of Problems   84
5.1   Ceremonies Performed for Patients With Seizures,
      Controls, and Depressed Patients   92
5.2   The Usc of the Evilway Sings   93
5.3   Use of Physicians and Ceremonial Practitioners
      for Self–Defined Illness   96
5.4   Patients Who Received Ceremonial Treatments
      Appropriate for Their Seizures   97
5.5   Treatment of Epileptics and Hysterics With
      Seizure-Specific Sings   98
5.6   Social Problems of Female Epileptics and
      Hysterics   99
5.7   Incest, Rape, and/or Illegitimate Children Among
      Female Epileptics   99
8.1   Sibling and Clan Incest in the Tuba City Service
      Unit   148

Acknowledgments

The research on which this book is based originated as a joint venture with Dr. Bert Kaplan, University of California, Santa Cruz. Dr. Kaplan's support made Neutra's participation during the summer of 1964 possible. Others whose participation was supported by Dr. Kaplan during that first summer's fieldwork were Dr. David Gutmann, Dr. Richard Randolph, and Wilson Wheatcroft; and interpreters Mrs. Margaret José, Mr. Max Hanley, and Mr. Howard McKinley, Jr. We wish to thank all of these coworkers for their contributions to the research effort. We are especially grateful for Dr. Kaplan's imaginative and stimulating encouragement.

We are also indebted to Dr. Charles S. MacCammon, then Director of the Navajo Area Office, Indian Health Service, for his support and cooperation. Dr. George Bock, then Chief of Medical Services for the Navajo Area, guided the evaluation of the medical records. His expertise and cooperation are appreciated.

A National Institute of Mental Health Career Development Award (#5-K3-MH-31,181; 1966–1971) made it possible for Levy to maintain contact with the patients during much of the follow-up phase of the research.

Between 1966 and 1975, Dr. Robert Bergman, then Director of Mental Health Programs of the Indian Health Service, took an active interest in the research and made it possible for Parker, as a Mental Health Technician, to maintain contact with the patients in the Tuba City Service Unit. Dr. John Porvasnik, Director of the Tuba City Service Unit, supported the final review and evaluation of all patients' charts.

Dr. Francis McNaughton (McGill University) reviewed and commented on the case studies. Dr. David F. Aberle (University of British Columbia), Dr. Stephen J. Kunitz (University of Rochester), and Dr. Arthur Kleinman (Harvard University) read and commented on an early draft.

The epidemiological survey was conducted under the auspices of the Indian Children's Program of the Indian Health Service. We are especially grateful for the support and advice provided by Dr. Al Hiat, Program Director, and Dr. Bill Douglas of the Indian Health Service Mental Health Program.

The survey was begun at Zuni thanks in large part to the initiative taken by Mr. Stanley Ghachu (Mental Health Technician, IHS), who made it possible for Levy to work freely in the community and who served as guide and mentor, helping to review charts and conduct interviews. His friendship and dedication made life at Zuni memorable. During this phase of the research, Levy was supported by a grant from the Epilepsy Foundation of America.

The chart reviews and interviews among the Tewa Pueblos were conducted by Dr. LeMyra DeBruyn, Miss Tessie Naranjo, and Anthony Archeuleta (Mental Health Technician, IHS). We thank them for their enthusiasm and persistence.

The work at Hopi was made possible by the assistance of Dr. Chuck North (Field Medical Officer, Keams Canyon Hospital), and Mrs. Betty Polingyumptewa (Director of Field Health Nursing). Dr. Eric Henderson shared the tasks of interviewing and of reviewing charts for the Hopi and Tuba City patients.

Without the cooperation of the many patients and their families, the research could not have been undertaken. Though they must remain anonymous, we extend to them our appreciation for their cooperation and forbearance and express the hope that in some way, the findings of this study will contribute to better understanding and improved services.

CHAPTER 1

Introduction

Epilepsy is a universal affliction and an awesome phenomenon. The suddenness of its appearance and the inexorable quality of its progression make clear to all that it is one of those facts of nature whose presence cannot be altered but which, in some manner, must be accounted for and incorporated into the fabric of life. The Greeks called it the sacred disease, believing that the victim was possessed by the gods. The Navajo Indians believe that sibling incest produces the signs of the major epileptic seizure (Haile 1978; Levy, Neutra, and Parker 1979). The transgressor of this important tabu, like the moth from which the disease takes its name, twists, convulses, and, in so doing, is likely to fall into the fire. This Navajo disease, called "moth madness," creates a role for the patient that is entirely disvalued. The healing ceremony, Mothway, is one of the most dangerous and powerful of all Navajo ceremonies. Its practitioners are themselves suspected of being witches because good men fear to become intimate with such dangerous powers.

Signs and symptoms very much like those of complex partial (psychomotor) seizures are thought to be caused by a particular form of witchcraft which has been translated variously as prostitution, excess, and frenzy witchcraft (Haile 1978; Kluckhohn 1962:37–41, 182, 230; Wyman and Kluckhohn 1938:5). The essential qualities of the epileptic psychomotor seizure are an alteration of consciousness and various simple, as well as complex, purposeful, automatic behaviors. Paroxysms among some patients can involve psychotic behavior or hallucinations and illusory perceptions of the various sensory systems. The Navajos believe that young women are the special victims, as they are the targets of witches who seek to seduce them. The victim, in a typical description, utters a brief cry, runs about aimlessly or in circles, and is likely to tear off her clothing and to disappear into the night before sinking into unconciousness.

Frenzy witchcraft is used primarily to seduce young women but may also be used to win at gambling or to ensure success on the hunt.

"Hand trembling" is the dominant mode of diagnosing illness, locating lost objects, and identifying witches. As described by Navajos, it resembles the simple partial seizures that involve the unilateral trembling of an extremity. The person whose arm trembles or shakes uncontrollably is thought to be possessed by the spirit of the supernatural Gila Monster and to be gifted with powers of divination (Wyman 1936a; 1936b). If the ceremony that initiates the person into the role of hand trembler is not performed, the seizures will become uncontrollable and will then be defined as an illness and not as a gift.

This book is concerned, first of all, with discovering why the Navajos have accorded seizures such importance, why sibling incest is associated with epilepsy, and what meaning this has in the larger context of Navajo culture. A second line of inquiry explores how and to what extent Navajos actually discriminate among seizures, whether epileptics are distinguished from hysterics with pseudoseizures, whether epileptics are chosen to become diagnosticians, and whether hysterics actually emulate the culturally defined signs of possession by Gila Monster.

In the Western World, epilepsy has occupied a crucial role in the long battle between magic and scientific conceptions of disease because it exhibits psychic as well as physical symptoms, thus lending itself to both supernatural and physiological interpretations (Temkin 1971:3). This, and the fact that hysteria, a psychological disorder, may take the form of pseudoseizures make it possible to explore the kinds of dichotomies utilized by a magico-religious healing system like that of the Navajo for the purpose of disease classification. The large gulf that separates modern Western medicine from traditional Navajo beliefs notwithstanding, the major epileptic seizure is a phenomenon both societies can recognize and discuss on the basis of its signs and symptoms alone. This area of agreement is no more than that. It does not imply that Navajos distinguish epilepsy from other seizure disorders with any accuracy. Nor do we wish to convey the idea that epilepsy presents no problems to the physician. Not only are there several different types of epileptic seizures, but similar seizures may be organically based, like epilepsy, or of psychic origin, as when conversion hysteria takes the form of pseudoseizures. It is, in consequence, often difficult for the physician to make an accurate diagnosis. Still, it is the very fact that seizures result from a number of causes and are varied in their manifestations that allows us to investigate the degree to which a society such as the Navajos' discriminates among them.

Regardless of the postulated causes of seizures, whether they are thought to be due to possession by an evil spirit or to supernatural punishment for breach of tabu, the signs of the major epileptic seizure are accurately described in some of the earliest written records. An ancient Akkadian text mentions a person whose neck turns to the side, whose hands and feet are tense, whose eyes are staring, and who froths at the mouth and loses consciousness (Temkin 1971:3–4). In the New Testament (Mark 9:17–22), Jesus is presented with a man who falls to the ground, gnashes his teeth, and foams at the mouth. The condition had persisted since the man's childhood and had often caused him to fall into fires or into bodies of water, thus endangering his life. It is important to determine the degree to which the accurate observation of seizures is the basis on which a prescientific society classifies various seizure disorders because magical notions of causation may just as easily lead to sorting patients into groups that do not correspond to the categories recognized by modern medicine.

Attention has been drawn to the fact that, in cultures other than our own, psychotherapy is marked by a unity of the medical, the psychological, and the spiritual (Price-Williams 1975:87). In marked contrast, it is said, our own medical system attempts to distinguish the mental from the physical, intellect from emotion, and abstract from concrete modes of thought (Price-Williams 1975:27, 31). The Navajos class illnesses by supernatural cause rather than by signs and symptoms. Diagnosis identifies the causal agent, which is then removed by the appropriate ceremony. By investigating actual patients as opposed to relying solely on normative statements elicited from knowledgeable informants, we will explore the possibility that the Navajo process of diagnosis and treatment utilizes a system which is perhaps less explicit than the one used to class diseases but which does, in fact, make discriminations much like those made in our own society.

The ability of the hysteric to fabricate symptoms that have symbolic meaning and the contrasting immutability of the epileptic convulsion together provide an opportunity to investigate several ideas concerning the relationship between culture and psychopathology which have engaged the interest of anthropologists for some years. Ever since Freud's theories of personality development and the genesis of neuroses became widely known in the United States, many anthropologists have held the view that psychopathologies are largely shaped by cultural conditioning. Some have asserted that the psychoses as well as the neuroses are environmentally determined, and the concept of the "culture bound" psychosis or "syndrome" has received much attention in the literature. Such phenomena are thought to arise when various features of the culture create unique personalities or exert unusual stresses on individuals and, in consequence, create psychic symptoms which are not found anywhere else. *Windigo,* an aberrant behavior said to have been found among the Ojibwa Indians, has been described as a "clearly localized psychosis" (Linton 1956:65). Other mental states, such as *latah, pibloctoq,* and arctic hysteria have been classed as culture-specific anxiety states and hysterias (Foulkes 1972; H. B. M. Murphy, 1976; Teicher 1960).

Ruth Benedict, in her widely read book, "Patterns of Culture," postulated that, although various signs and symptoms may occur across cultures, societies are free to label them as normal or abnormal in a somewhat arbitrary manner:

It is clear that culture may value and make socially acceptable even highly unstable human types. If it chooses to treat their peculiarities as the most valued variants of human behavior, the individuals in question will rise to the occasion and perform their social roles without reference to our usual ideas of the types who can make social adjustments and those who cannot. Those who function inadequately in any society are not those with certain fixed "abnormal" traits, but may well be those whose responses have received no support in the institutions of their culture." (Benedict 1960:229–33)

Benedict believed that not only transient episodes of trance but also seizures and long periods of violent insanity were honored in many societies. More recently, it has been suggested that the only significant difference between acute schizophrenics and shamans is the degree to which society accepts and provides a social role for the person who displays the signs and symptoms of schizophrenia (Silverman 1967). Although most anthropologists who have published on the subject have taken a more cautious position, the idea that a set of behaviors, which, in our society, would be labeled as psychotic, can be labeled as normal or even valued by another society is an intriguing one which has not been thoroughly investigated.

There is also interest in the efficacy of non-Western forms of treatment. Magical treatments are thought by many to alleviate psychic distress. As eminent an anthropologist as Claude Lévi-Strauss has asserted that Cuna women experiencing a difficult childbirth have their ordeal made easier by the ministrations of a shaman who recites a myth text symbolically representing the descent of the newborn through the birth canal (Lévi-Strauss 1963:186–205). Others have maintained that the very act of becoming a shaman, a healer who attains his position by having a mystical experience and by exhibiting psychotic behavior, is itself a therapeutic process that cures the psychotic (Silverman 1967).

Would Navajo epileptics with unilateral partial seizures actually be chosen to perform as hand-trembler diagnosticians? Would it even be possible for hysterical patients who displayed unilateral pseudoseizures to perform the role adequately? Or is the professional Navajo diagnostician an individual who is normal by modern medical standards but who is able to attain a state during which the hand or arm shakes without seeming to be consciously controlled?

If hysterical pseudoseizures are almost infinitely malleable, one would expect Navajo conversion hysterias to look like hand trembling in most cases because this form of seizure is positively valued and the individual can gain attention by imitating it. Conversely, pseudoseizures resembling the major epileptic seizure should occur less frequently because of the belief that they are caused by incest, so that all the hysteric could expect to gain would be rejection. The question also arises whether individuals who have committed sibling incest develop hysterical pseudoseizures. Further, would epileptics develop hysterical symptoms as a consequence of social stigmatization or do the healing ceremonies provide a degree of support sufficient to avoid undue psychological stress?

The condition produced by frenzy witchcraft is thought to be relatively transient. A young, hysterical woman with sexual problems might find ample room for acting-out behavior, as well as rewarding attention without censure, by emulating this form of seizure—especially in light of the fact that the ceremonial cure utilizes datura, a plant with hallucinogenic properties. Epileptics with complex partial seizures might easily be diagnosed as suffering from frenzy witchcraft, but we thought it unlikely that their seizures would be ameliorated by the ceremony.

None of the ideas about the influence of culture on psychiatric disorders has gone unchallenged. Most descriptions of non-Western psychopathologies are anecdotal descriptions of small groups of cases with no relation to a standard population (Lemkau and Crocetti 1958). Most of the studies that attempt to calculate prevalence rates are based upon hospitalized populations which reflect neither a true incidence nor a true profile of the different symptoms in the societies studied (P. K. Benedict 1958). Many societies are apt to be more "hospitable" to some symptoms than to others, and many still find modern medicine to be an intrusive institution and, consequently, do not utilize it in a manner comparable to Western populations. For these reasons, hospital behavior may differ appreciably from home behavior, and even the presenting symptoms may be carefully selected when the hospital is utilized. In addition, psychopathologies among primitive peoples tend to be poorly defined in terms of Western systems of classification. But whether this is due to the existence of different forms of mental illness in different societies, to the limitations of Western taxonomies themselves, or to the difficulties involved in observing symptoms in unfamiliar societies is not clear.

The difficulties involved in making diagnoses in prescientific societies are many (Wallace 1964:164–98). Functional psychoses are almost impossible to distinguish from organically based ones in areas not served by well-equipped hospitals. It is also generally the case that research in such areas is more likely to be undertaken by anthropologists than by neurologists or psychiatrists, and many valuable anthropological insights tend to be invalidated by the anthropologists' limited clinical awareness and knowledge of the broader fields of genetics and medicine (P. K. Benedict 1958:727). The signs, symptoms, and progression of the major seizures of epilepsy, on the other hand, are agreed upon by physicians, and differential diagnosis is made more secure by the use of an electroencephalograph, which amplifies and displays changes in what are called brain waves, the electrical activity of the most superficial layers of the brain.

The Navajos comprise the largest tribe of Indians in the United States. Currently with a population over 150,000, they occupy a reservation in northern Arizona, New Mexico, and southern Utah which is approximately the size of the state of West Virginia. Placed on a reservation in 1868, they have retained much of their traditional religion despite considerable changes in their economic and political organization and exposure to extensive Christian missionizing. This retention of a precontact religion, together with the fact that the U.S. Public Health Service provides comprehensive health care for the Navajos and other tribes in the region, makes the reservation an almost ideal area in which to investigate traditional medical systems. The task of calibrating modern medical and Navajo categories is furthered by the fact that most Navajos rely on Western medicine about as much as they do on the older ceremonial system. Thus, a cohort of patients diagnosed by physicians can be studied to determine the extent to which the native distinctions agree with or diverge from those used by modern physicians.

The meanings that seizures have for the Navajos and the reasons for them can only be approached in the broader context of Navajo history and religion; it is to this context that we now turn our attention. The Navajos' Athabascan-speaking ancestors entered the Southwest sometime between 1300 and

1525 (Brugge 1983). By 1630, the Navajos were doing some
farming and had frequent contact with the Pueblos. Other
Athabascan speakers occupied areas to the south and east of
what was to become known as Navajo country and, over time,
became distinct tribes known today as Apaches. Among these,
the Western Apaches are closest to the Navajos with respect to
reliance on agriculture and the development of matrilineal descent groups. Unlike the Navajos, however, none of the Apaches
ever became pastoralists prior to the reservation period.

Intensive interaction of the Navajos with various Pueblo
groups began in 1690, when the Spaniards reconquered the area
after the Pueblo Revolt of 1680, and lasted until about 1770.
Tewa, Jemez, Keresan, Zuni, and Hopi refugees lived among the
Navajos during this period. According to Brugge, Navajo religion and social life became Puebloized at this time. Navajos
adopted Pueblo architectural styles, techniques of manufac-
ture, religious paraphernalia, and many elements of nonma-
terial culture.

After 1770, drought, intensified Ute raiding, and a resump-
tion of warfare with the Spaniards led to a migration of the
Navajos to the south and west of their center of settlement in
the upper San Juan River drainage. The pueblito settlements
were abandoned, and the population became more dispersed.[1]
Presumably farming declined somewhat in importance at this
time as well, and Pueblo elements of social and religious organization became increasingly more diluted. By the early 1800s,
stockraising had become as important as agriculture and, during the early years of the reservation period, it became the
dominant subsistence pursuit.

Several authors interpret the development of Navajo religion
as an attempt to incorporate the communal values borrowed
from the Pueblos into the persisting, individualistic orienta-
tion of the original hunting and gathering world view of the
early Athabascan immigrants. Brugge, for example, believes
that the Blessingway ceremonial began to assume its contemporary form as "the core of a nativistic reassertion of the
Athabascan way of life" and that "Blessingway holds a central
position in Navajo religion and the Navajo way of life, giving
both a unity in spite of a complex diversity" (Brugge 1963:22,

25). Similarly, Luckert (1975: chaps. 7–8; 1979:3–12) sees the trickster figure, Coyote, as the symbol of the surviving element of an archaic shamanism which is in conflict with Pueblo traditions.

Bert Kaplan and Dale Johnson (1964) have speculated about the behavioral consequences of this conflict between the two traditions: the one a concern for personal and magical "power," the other for maintenance of social control and harmony. Over time, according to these authors, the Pueblo tradition came to dominate, so that, in the present era, with hunting and raiding almost extinct, there are no vital institutions for the expression of the early Athabascan tradition. Athabascan values, however, have not disappeared but have been repressed, finding their expression in patterns of deviance and psychopathology.

The belief that disease is caused by possession of the soul by a malevolent force is common among the hunting and gathering tribes of North America. Kaplan and Johnson believe that "it is in this notion of possession, subtle and vaguely stated though it is, that the core of Navajo conceptions of mental illness is to be found. . . . attributing illness to a power that possesses one, whether a devil or unconsciousness, rather than to oneself, is the typical mechanism of hysterical illness" (Kaplan and Johnson 1964:206). Without claiming that hysteria is common among the Navajos, they do believe that the most characteristic Navajo illnesses have, as a central element, abdication of ego control. The most prevalent type of Navajo psychopathology they have called "crazy violence" or "crazy drunken violence," which is not only hysterical but also an attack on normal social arrangements—in other words, an expression of the repressed Athabascan traits. This attempt to infer personality traits from cultural beliefs is an elaboration of Ruth Benedict's characterization of the cultures of North America:

The basic contrast between the Pueblos and the other cultures of North America is the contrast that is named and described by Nietzsche in his studies of Greek tragedy. He discusses two diametrically opposed ways of arriving at the value of existence. The Dionysian pursues them through "the annihilation of the ordinary bounds and limits of existence"; he seeks to attain in his most valued moments escape from the boundaries imposed upon him by his five senses, to break through into another order of experience. The desire of the Dionysian, in personal experience or in ritual, is to press through it toward a certain psychological state, to achieve excess. The closest analogy to the emotions he seeks is drunkenness, and he values the illuminations of frenzy. . . . The Apollonian distrusts all this, and has often little idea of the nature of such experiences. He finds means to outlaw them from his conscious life. He "knows but one law, measure in the Hellenic sense." He keeps the middle of the road, stays within the known map, does not meddle with disruptive psychological states. . . . even in the exaltation of the dance he "remains what he is, and retains his civic name." (Benedict 1960:79–80)

If Dionysian personality traits persist in Navajo culture, and disease is thought to be caused by possession, we would expect a greater prevalence of hysterical disorders among the Navajos than the Pueblos. One might also hypothesize that the symptoms of hysteria should prove to be more flamboyant than those exhibited by the Apollonian Pueblos. The Navajos should also resemble their linguistic and cultural congeners, the Apaches, more closely than the Pueblos because they share a common pre-agricultural past and because the Apaches interacted less intensely with the Pueblos than did the Navajos. If this interpretation is correct, seizures and other dissociative states should have cultural meaning for the Apaches as well as for the Navajos.

There are, however, reasons to believe that this may not be the case. First, a number of studies have shown that, although most Indian tribes have high rates of suicide, homicide, and alcoholism, the Navajos appear more like the Pueblos in this regard, with similar homicide and suicide rates and rather lower rates of alcoholic cirrhosis than the Pueblos (Levy and Kunitz 1971, 1974; Levy, Kunitz, and Henderson in press; Van Winkle and May 1986). If the Navajos are more Apollonian than Dionysian, hysterical disorders and beliefs about disease causation should not differ much among Navajos and various Pueblo tribes, and specifically Navajo beliefs about seizures must be accounted for without recourse to general personality traits alone. Second, the interpretation of Navajo religion and values here described neglects more than a century of pastoralism, implying, in effect, that no value conflicts developed as a consequence of this major shift in subsistence pursuits. In the chapters that follow we will develop the argument that the Navajos' preoccupation with seizures and incest is the result of historical developments that took place after 1770 and that have no counterparts among either the Apaches or the Pueblos. Without denying that there may have been a conflict between individualistic Dionysian and communal Apollonian values during the period when Navajos and Pueblos lived together, we shall propose (a) that current Navajo interpretations of the incest tabu developed after they became pastoral seminomads and (b) that the preoccupation with incest and seizures is peculiar to the Navajos and is consequent on social tensions stemming directly from the shift to pastoralism.

The Course of the Research

The research on which this study is based is of two types. The first is a detailed study of a cohort of patients diagnosed in Indian Health Service hospitals as either epileptic or hysterical. Special attention was paid to their seizure histories, traditional diagnoses, and ceremonial treatments. The second is an epidemiological survey of epilepsy and hysteria among the Navajos, Hopis, Zunis, and Tewas.

In 1964, diagnosed epileptics and hysterics living in the Tuba City and Fort Defiance Service Units were identified by reviewing all admissions to the hospitals serving those areas. The Tuba City Service Unit comprised the westernmost portion of the reservation. The Navajos of this area were, at that time, thought to be more traditional and less reliant on wage work than residents of the Fort Defiance Service Unit. The Tuba City area is about the size of the state of Rhode Island and, during the 1930s, there was less than one person per square mile as compared to a population density of approximately two and a half persons in the Fort Defiance area. This latter Service Unit, located in the eastern half of the reservation, has had a longer history of contact with Spaniards and Anglo Americans and more exposure to wage work. Fort Defiance was the center of the original 1868 reservation, and today Window Rock, some 6 miles away, serves as the governmental and administrative center of the reservation. These contrasting areas were selected because we thought it likely that traditional health beliefs and practices might have changed more radically in the Fort Defiance area. In the event, no measurable differences were discerned and thus areal differences need not be considered further.

Sixty-nine patients were identified by this method. After reviewing the medical charts and discarding mistakes in coding, epileptic children under six years of age, and retarded children who had been institutionalized, forty individuals—nineteen from Tuba City and twenty-one from Fort Defiance—were selected for study.

The medical staffs of the two hospitals reviewed the charts with us to assess the reliability of the recorded diagnoses. Thirty of these patients and their immediate families were interviewed in their homes. Ten were given a lower priority because they were either children still under twelve years of age or alcoholics who had developed seizures subsequent to their drinking later in life. The field interviews obtained a life history, a full description of the symptoms, and a history of Navajo diagnoses and ceremonial treatments. A psychologist, Dr. David Gutman of the University of Michigan, was able to interview several individuals with hysterical seizures and to administer a projective test, the Thematic Apperception Test. A number of patients with poor seizure descriptions and histories in their medical charts were more accurately diagnosed. With the new information thus obtained, physicians in the hospital were able to locate a number of missing electroencephalograph reports during the summer, which also improved diagnostic accuracy.

We compared the ceremonies performed for the seizure patients with those performed for individuals already studied by Levy from 1959 through 1964 to see whether they differed in any significant way. These people were from two areas typical of the Tuba City area. One was a group of kinsmen of all ages, numbering about 100, who were rural pastoralists living about 30 miles from the hospital. The second, also comprised of about 100 people of all ages, were from randomly selected families living adjacent to the government compound of Tuba City.

These families relied more on wage work or social welfare and were, on average, more acculturated. The health status and hospital-use patterns of these two groups had already been studied, and it was known that their disease profile approximated that of the tribe as a whole.

During the field interviews, families and knowledgeable individuals living in one community within the Tuba City Service Unit were asked whether they knew anyone with seizures. The purpose of this procedure was to determine whether the case-finding procedure missed a significant number of epileptics. In the event, all individuals identified in this manner were either found not to have epilepsy or to be epileptics who had been diagnosed while away in boarding school. At the same time we made an effort to identify all individuals thought to have committed sibling incest in this community to see whether there was any real association with seizures.

Between 1965 and 1975, we were able to spend several weeks each summer contacting the patients who lived in the Tuba City Service Unit, as well as some individuals with a variety of medical conditions who had been identified either in the community or by Navajo hospital personnel as having "spells." Interviews with these people allowed us to see just how often those who did not have seizures were really thought to have them. We were also able to see whether the diagnoses and treatments given to these individuals were the same as those given to the epileptics. During the same period, an Indian Health Service psychiatrist was able to evaluate two patients whose psychiatric symptoms presented diagnostic problems, and the internists in Tuba City were able to get added electroencephalograms from two of the patients whose seizures were the most difficult to diagnose.

In 1975, the medical charts were reviewed and everyone in the original study group who lived in the Tuba City Service Unit was reinterviewed. This enabled us to compare the careers of epileptics with those of the patients with hysterical pseudoseizures over the period of a decade.

The reliability of information gained through survey techniques is always open to question when the subject of inquiry is sensitive or the respondents are of another culture and speak

English imperfectly, if at all. That Parker, a seasoned medical interpreter, was a Navajo from one of the areas studied and that he and Levy were well known in that area we knew would be in our favor. We had not anticipated that our identification with the Indian Health Service would be viewed as positively as it was, however. Neutra and the less experienced interpreters hired in the Fort Defiance area had little difficulty gaining the cooperation necessary to conduct detailed interviews. The reaction most often expressed was that it was "about time" the Health Service took an interest in this problem and that it was a pleasant surprise to see White physicians actually visiting families in their homes.

By 1975, it was apparent that a more thorough epidemiological survey was necessary if the prevalence of epilepsy was to be accurately assessed. Moreover, it had become painfully clear that it would not be possible to determine whether Navajos had a high prevalence of hysterical disorders or whether Navajo epileptics had more psychological problems as a consequence of negative beliefs about the disorder unless controlled comparisons could be made with populations who did not hold these beliefs. The Navajos could not be compared with the general U.S. population because pseudoseizures and the psychological problems faced by epileptics, though frequently described in books on the subject, have rarely been studied by epidemiologists.

By 1977, the Indian Health Service had computerized its recording system so that it was possible to identify individuals from Zuni, Hopi, the Tewa-speaking Pueblos, and the Navajos of the Tuba City Service Unit who had been diagnosed as having epilepsy, any hysterical disorder, or seizures of any variety. Patients seen as outpatients as well as those referred to facilities outside the federal system on a contract basis were included in the data bank along with those seen and diagnosed in Indian Health Service Hospitals.

At the present time, the Zunis live on a reservation some 40 miles south of Gallup, New Mexico. They are served by an Indian Health Service hospital located 5 miles from their main village as well as by the larger IHS hospital in Gallup. The five Tewa-speaking Pueblo villages are located approximately 25 miles north of Sante Fé, New Mexico, and use the government hospital in that city. The Hopi reservation is surrounded by that of the Navajo in Arizona. They are served by a hospital on their own reservation as well as by the one in Tuba City. The surveys were conducted between 1978 and 1980.

Presentation

Chapters 2 and 3 discuss Navajo disease theory, healing practices, and the meanings Navajos have given to the various seizures and mental states in the myths that recount their origins and supernatural cures. Because the Navajos entered the Southwest as hunters and gatherers and only developed their present system of beliefs after sustained contact with the Pueblo inhabitants of the area, Navajo health culture is placed in a comparative context. The shamanistic practices of most North American hunting and gathering tribes are contrasted with the religions of the sedentary Pueblos. Many direct borrowings from the Pueblos are found in the Navajo myths. In Chapter 2 the general structure of the Navajo ceremonial system is compared with that of the Pueblos. Navajo disease theory and ceremonialism are patterned after Pueblo models, especially Hopi. As among the Hopis, possession is not thought to be a cause of disease and the shamanistic sucking cure and diagnosing by hand trembling are relatively recent borrowings from the Apaches. Coyote, the trickster creator god of the hunters and gatherers, has been demoted by the Navajos to a symbol of evil.

Chapter 3 examines Pueblo and Navajo beliefs about seizures and the myth traditions on which they are based. Seizures are placed in a larger class of disorders involving irrational and extreme behaviors thought to derive from the irrational excesses of Coyote, which are usually of a sexual nature. Yet the myths explaining the origins of moth madness and frenzy witchcraft are Pueblo. The association with Coyote is made with only minimal mythic elements, suggesting that these illnesses do not represent earlier shamanistic themes. The association of sibling incest with seizures is unique to the Navajos and is found neither among the Pueblos nor among the

Apaches. A question raised but not answered is why father-daughter incest is not thought to cause a specific disease and is not given so salient a position in Navajo mythology as is sibling incest.

Because only the medically oriented reader is well informed on the subject of seizure disorders, the presentation of the epidemiological data in Chapter 4 is preceded by a discussion of how scientific medicine currently defines, classifies, and diagnoses the various forms of epilepsy and pseudoseizures of psychic origin. Our diagnostic criteria are also presented in this chapter. We also present the epidemiological distribution of seizures among the four Indian tribes. In this way the reader may become familiar with the "medical reality" before attempting to see the world through Navajo eyes. The possibility that a high prevalence of epilepsy among the Navajos led to a heightened concern with seizures is discounted as the Navajo rate is identical with those of the various Pueblo groups. The prevalence of hysteria among the Navajos is not higher than is reported for other populations and, although it is higher than that of the Pueblos, the difference is due to the fact that Navajo epileptics tend to have more psychological problems than Pueblo epileptics and not to a general tendency to hysteria as postulated by Kaplan and Johnson.

The degree to which Navajos successfully discriminate between generalized and partial seizures, epileptic and pseudoseizures, and among seizures and other disorders is assessed in Chapter 5. Individuals with seizures received diagnoses and ceremonial treatments that distinguished them from clinically depressed patients as well as from patients with a variety of more common disorders. Hysterics were also treated differently from epileptics and had fewer social and psychological problems. The discrimination is made possible because epilepsy is more chronic and debilitating than is hysteria.

Chapters 6, 7, and 8 examine hand trembling, frenzy witchcraft, and moth madness in some detail. The careers of epileptics and hysterics are compared, and the association of generalized seizures with incest, complex partial seizures with frenzy witchcraft, and simple partial (unilateral) seizures with hand trembling is examined. No epileptics were thought to be qualified to become hand tremblers. Although some hysterics presented their symptoms as unilateral trembling, the only individuals selected to become diagnosticians were the daughters of hand tremblers. Hysterics were not able to perform the role successfully, and their symptoms were not alleviated by either the healing ceremonies or the performance of the diagnostic trance state.

Most of the hysterics had spells that looked like psychomotor seizures and were diagnosed as suffering from frenzy witchcraft. Although these patients were treated for frenzy witchcraft, love magic and seduction were not included in the accounts. Instead the witches were said to be trying to kill their victims. Fathers were sometimes identified as the witch, and several women were attempting to free themselves from domineering and authoritative fathers. These findings raise further questions about father-daughter incest: whether it is as much a cause of concern as sibling incest, why it is not thought to cause a specific illness, and whether frenzy witchcraft has come to serve de facto as the disease which embraces problems arising from disturbed father-daughter relationships.

Epileptics with generalized seizures were thought to have committed incest; therefore, they suffered considerable stigmatization. The postulated link between seizures and incest actually creates a self-fulfilling prophecy, as several epileptics were seduced by siblings, real and classificatory, after the onset of their seizures.

Chapter 9 identifies what we believe to be the primary reasons for the Navajos' preoccupation with seizures and proffers our reconstruction of the history of Navajo belief about incest and sexual witchcraft. We argue that rules against marriage into own clan and clan group, father's clan, and mother's father's clan developed during the period of Puebloization, during which large numbers of Pueblo descent groups had to be integrated into the Navajo polity. Clan endogamy in all its forms became the cause of serious disease at this time. Later, during the period of pastoralism, concerns with familial incest were heightened as the population became dispersed, and families lived in isolation until the rule against endogamy came to be seen as applying to siblings and clan siblings exclusively. These developments were unique to the Navajos and explain the association of seizures with incest. They do not, however, indicate that the Navajos had a greater involvement with incest than other tribes, especially the Apaches whom they resemble in many respects. Nor is the idea that Navajos have a predilection for hysterical reactions confirmed by these data.

CHAPTER 2

The Healing Tradition

Over the course of time, the simple hunting and gathering society of the early Navajos was transformed into one of greater complexity—more like that of the agricultural Pueblos into whose area they had penetrated. Authors describing the ceremonial patterns of the southwestern culture area have emphasized the contrasts between the Dionysian shamanism of the hunters and gatherers and the communal values of the Apollonian Pueblos despite the fact that both were built on a common foundation of belief about the nature of supernatural power and the causes of disease (Underhill 1948; Lamphere 1983). Before the development of Pueblo religion and subsequent Navajo adaptations can be traced, it is therefore necessary to consider shamanistic belief and practices.

Shamanism

Throughout North America people prayed to animals before killing them, avoided beings and objects thought to cause disease, and attempted to control supernatural power. Indeed, a list of the beliefs and practices of one tribe alone is both long and seemingly devoid of organizational logic. More puzzling still is the qualitative equivalence given to humans, animals, and all aspects of the natural environment: men and animals assume each other's outer forms, and the inanimate is animate. The concepts that give coherence to the cosmology are those of supernatural power, the soul, and the evolution of life forms.

No creation myths have been recorded for many hunting and gathering peoples who may never, in fact, have troubled themselves with the question of ultimate origins. Where such accounts do exist, however, a formless universe is shaped and given life by one or more creators. Supernatural power was the animating force placed into all beings who helped the creator shape the world. During the mythic "first times" there was no difference in the outer forms of these beings. Gradually, however, differentiation took place, and from some of these primordial beings are descended the creatures of the present world. Some retained their original supernatural essence intact, while others were placed in such inanimate forms as the sun, moon, and stars. Thus, in the present world, when a human wished to kill an animal, he remembered that it was a "child" of a particular primordial supernatural and offered prayers so that its ancestor spirit would not be offended.

Although mythic humans with supernatural powers existed in the beginning of creation, in the present world humankind stood somewhat apart. The souls of animals returned to their spirit ancestor to be born again, but the souls of men went to an underworld from which they could not return. Animals seemed to live their lives passively, exercising little volition; humans, however, had always to guard against the threat to life posed by uncontrolled power. The primordial supernaturals continued to dwell in the world above but could descend to earth or the underworld at will; humans remained on earth.

Survival among hunting and gathering peoples required success in the hunt and protection from sickness and death. In consequence, the individual was of paramount importance and rituals dealt almost exclusively with these concerns. In some tribes, notably those of the Plains, all men and many women actively sought power by means of a vision quest. For the majority of tribes, however, the average person either attained little power or none at all and had to rely on those rare individuals who did—the shamans.

The quintessential North American shaman was someone who received power from one or more spirit helpers during a vision experience and who effected cures by communicating with these supernaturals while in a trance. It was the trance that distinguished the shaman from the ceremonialist, or priest. The intensity of the trance experience varied among tribes. Violent dissociative states involving spasmodic convulsions and other forms of motor hyperexcitement were common. Among the Shoshoneans of the Great Basin, on the other hand, individuals received supernatural powers over a number of years through dreams which started during childhood. Of itself, power was neither good nor evil but could be used for harmful as well as constructive purposes; because shamans controlled large amounts of it, they were often feared. Witches were those individuals who preferred to use power to destroy others, so that shamans were suspected of being witches as often as they were respected for their curing powers. Witchcraft accusations and the fear of being accused deterred shamans from becoming too wealthy and powerful in what were essentially egalitarian societies.

Disease theory held that sickness was caused by intrusive objects, loss or possession of the soul, and violation of tabus. Witches, malevolent supernaturals, or chance alone could cause a foreign object to enter a victim and cause sickness. The cure was accomplished by "sucking" the intrusive object from the body. Although superficial lacerations were sometimes made, usually no bodily damage was done. The shaman, who had hidden some small object—a stone, bird claw, or arrow point—in his mouth would hold it up for all present to see that the evil had been successfully removed. This legerdemain and other far more dramatic acts have been offered as proofs that shamans were either charlatans or self-deluded naifs. Indians themselves often expressed skepticism about individual shamans without attacking the beliefs upon which shamanistic healing was based. Lévi-Strauss (1963:175–78) discusses the story, recorded by Franz Boas, of a Kwakiutl Indian who became a shaman for the express purpose of exposing the entire healing profession of his tribe. Instead, his many successes convinced him that the technique worked. To understand why, one must understand the principles of magic utilized by the "sucking" cure.

Magic is based on the assumption of impersonal supernatural power, some of which, we have seen, was a prerequisite for life itself. According to Sir James Frazer (1922), the general law of sympathetic magic is that things act on each other from a distance through some secret sympathy. It is supernatural power that effects the transmission of impulses from one to the other. This general law is utilized in two ways: by "imitative" and by "contagious" magic. Imitative magic is based on the principle that "like begets like." If a successful kill is imitated, the hunt will be a success. For this result to occur, however, the shaman must imbue the imitative act with the supernatural power that will then transmit "impulses" from the ritual hunt to the real hunt. "Contagious" magic is predicated on the idea that things which have once been in contact with each other will retain a shared essence even after being separated. A witch needs only some item from his intended victim—hair, nails, feces, or a piece of clothing—to do him harm, for what is done to the object in the witch's possession is done also to the victim. The object held in the shaman's mouth during the sucking cure is an imitation of the object in the patient's body. The shaman sucks his object and, in so doing, also sucks the cause of the disease out of the patient. Always, however, the more power the shaman commands the better the chance for success, because the intrusive object may be imbued with the power of the witch.

Sudden fright was thought to dislodge souls. Souls were also stolen by witches and malevolent supernaturals, or souls were lost when displaced by an intruding spirit. Souls of the deceased remained in the vicinity of the burial for a period of time before descending to the netherworld. During this time they were considered dangerous, and contact with them caused sickness. Belonging to neither world, they were anomalous and, therefore malevolent. For the sake of convenience rather than accuracy, we call them ghosts. Ghosts resisted leaving this world and wanted to take the living with them—that is, to steal their souls. This aim was facilitated when an encounter with a ghost caused sudden shock or fright, or the survivor might be enticed to follow the deceased to the underworld. Not only are Orpheus myths common, but personal accounts of dream journeys into the world of the dead are still told.

To recover a stolen or lost soul, the shaman went into a trance during which his soul traveled to the spirit world in search of the victim's soul. Most frequently, the shaman was accompanied on the journey by his spirit helper, as witches could only be destroyed by a greater power. The outcome was always in doubt, however, and after his return, the shaman was often weak and close to death himself.

To Westerners, breach of tabu implies transgression of the moral code, an act in and of itself evil and deserving punishment. But among the Indians of North America, disfavored actions did not bring divine retribution by virtue of their immorality. Supernatural power was impersonal and morally neutral. A thief might be punished by the community, but stealing was not considered a cause of illness. Behaviors that led to sickness were those that brought one in contact with a disease-causing object or which imitated a mythic episode that accounted for a disease. For example, all supernaturals were to be avoided or treated with ceremonial respect in the event contact was unavoidable. Because a coyote footprint was once connected with a specific coyote who itself was a "child" of the powerful supernatural Coyote, inadvertently stepping or defecating on the footprint caused sickness according to the principle of "contagious" magic. Underlying the notion of disease through contact, however, is the mechanism of possession, because Coyote (in the case just given) is always thought of as entering and possessing the person who comes too close to him. In consequence, the cure was the same as that used for soul loss or possession.

We have seen that survival among hunters and gatherers depended to a great extent on individual prowess, so that hunt magic and curing ceremonies predominated over group ceremonies. There is one aspect of life we have not covered, however, and that involves the degree to which hunting societies were preoccupied with randomness and chance.

No society exalts chaos. Order and predictability are the prerequisites of social stability. But accidents and unforeseen disasters permeated the lives of those hunting peoples who lived in resource-scarce areas or those with harsh climates. Although the hunter knew the ways of his prey, a sudden storm or a torn tendon could bring all his efforts to nothing. Unlike the sedentary farmers who tended to view chance as an evil that could be controlled, the hunter accepted it, lived with it, and even tried to ally himself with it. The mythic Creator of the hunters was a trickster figure: Raven on the northwest coast, a vague humanoid throughout much of the eastern subarctic, and Coyote in the Rocky Mountain and desert West. Paul Radin has characterized Trickster as:

at one and the same time creator and destroyer, giver and negator, he who dupes others and who is always duped himself. He wills nothing consciously. At all times he is constrained to behave as he does from impulses over which he has no control. He knows neither good nor evil yet he is responsible for both. He possesses no values, moral or social, is at the mercy of his passions and appetites. Yet through his actions all values come into being. (Radin 1972:xxiii)

The chaos Coyote represents is that which dwells within the individual as well as that found in the external world. Coyote scatters the heavenly bodies in the sky, so that there will be less order and predictability in the universe. His appearance is always unexpected, and he is governed by his uncontrolled passions rather than by reason and self-discipline. If men create gods in their own image, this trickster figure is the epitome of the Dionysian personality. If his creations are admirable, his excesses give cause for anxiety. The Mescalero Apaches recognized the coyote in themselves when they said "Coyote did it first. We follow in Coyote's footsteps" (Opler 1938:215).

Pueblo Developments

After agriculture spread throughout the Southwest, shamanism and the vision quest were gradually overlaid by annual fertility and rain-making ceremonies among the tribes most dependent on farming. The Hopis, of all the Pueblos, were the least reliant on shamanistic beliefs and cures and thus best exemplify the development of Apollonian values.

Hopi society grew out of a Great Basin desert culture similar to that of the linguistically related Shoshones and Paiutes. Gathering was as important as hunting among the tribes of this arid region where large game animals were few and, in consequence, not imbued with such dangerous powers as among other groups of hunters. For this reason, perhaps, shamans were not so feared as they were in other areas, and their powers came to them over a number of years in dreams rather than in dramatic trance states (Steward 1933:308, 312; B. B. Whiting 1950:29). It seems likely that the transition was easier for the Hopis than for the other Pueblos because they did not have to overcome a very strong tradition of shamanism.

Typical Hopi healers were not true shamans because they did not utilize trance states, have spirit quests, or believe that illness was caused by soul loss (Jorgensen 1980:500, 564, 569; Underhill 1948:37). They received their power in a variety of ways: through dreams, after vows made during the course of an illness, or through ascription of power by virtue of birth into the Badger clan (Titiev 1943; 1972:54, 66). A gift for healing, but not for shamanistic power, was also thought to belong to those who were twins in embryo but who were then twisted "into one" so that they were born as single individuals (Talayesva 1942:25).

The Hopis continued to believe that witchcraft and intrusion of foreign objects were major causes of disease. Unlike the other Pueblos, however, the Hopis did not believe that witches caused disease by stealing the souls of their victims. The idea of soul loss was confined to the belief that a witch must steal the soul of a relative to prolong his own life. Such an occurrence was, however, not thought to be a cause of disease and there was no treatment for it (Titiev 1943:549).

The Hopis also made a significant change in the conceptualization of disease caused by breach of tabu. This etiological factor may have been even more important than witchcraft. The priestly societies that controlled the all-important agricultural ceremonies also treated those illnesses caused by trespass on their secrets or paraphernalia, as well as similar conditions resulting from such natural causes as snake bites and lightning strikes. We have had occasion to mention that among hunters and gatherers there was no personal blame attached to the transgression of tabus, which were breached, as often as not, by accident. The Hopis, however, placed great emphasis on the patient's responsibility for his own condition. Bad thoughts, improper actions, disbelief, emotional imbalance, and anxiety were all thought to cause illness. This was related to the importance placed on breach of tabu as a cause of disease and the belief that everyone must actively promote life and community well-being by being strong and by thinking only good thoughts. The ability of witches to cause illness was recognized, but it was, and still is, believed that an individual is more susceptible to penetration by witch objects if his thoughts are not good or if he is depressed or worried. Good thoughts provide considerable resistance to witchcraft. Healers and family members urged the patient to tell his bad thoughts, to put them "in the open," and then to "throw them away" (Aitken 1930:372–73).

This emphasis on the responsibility of the individual is incompatible with ideas of soul loss and possession which imply that the patient is helpless in the face of forces over which he has no control. The Hopis recognized that witchcraft might cause insanity and other forms of irrational behavior, and, in theory, the insane were not responsible for their mad acts. In practice, however, the madman was feared and shunned in the same way a witch was feared (Titiev 1972:353–54). Where soul loss is an accepted belief, the patient places himself in the hands of the all-powerful shaman, who assumes responsibility to combat and defeat the witch. Titiev thought that Hopis' reluctance to seek treatment from a shaman was due to the belief that they were witches (Titiev 1943:552). We are convinced that belief in personal responsibility is equally important, especially as this same reluctance is seen when treatment is sought from other types of Hopi healers and from physicians. In fact, Hopis questioned on this subject asserted that older shamans of good reputation were never feared, although younger, less well-established healers of all types might be considered incompetent or thought to be charlatans.

By emphasizing breach of tabu, developing the notion of individual responsibility for his own actions, and assigning many healing functions to the priests of the ceremonial societies, the Hopis began to dichotomize the concept of supernatural power. Like other Shoshonean speakers, Hopis believed that supernatural power could be used for either good or evil. But, unlike such tribes as the Paiutes, Shoshones, Utes, and Comanches who made no linguistic distinction between the shaman and the witch, referring to both as "one who uses power," the Hopis referred to the powers of shamans and witches by different terms. The morpheme *tuu* means supernatural power among the Hopi, Southern Paiute, and the speakers of Takic languages—i.e., the southern California Shoshoneans. Among the Numic speakers, however, it means "to die." *Powa* also means supernatural power in Hopi, Southern and Northern Paiute, Shoshone, Bannock, Mono, and among some other speakers of the Numic subfamily of Uto-Aztecan. In Hopi, a witch is called *powaka* (bad power), but the individual healer, or shaman, is *tuuhikya*.[1]

All the good aspects of power have been assigned to the ceremonial realm of the priests—*powata* means purify or cure; *powalawu* means performing a ritual; and a ritual song is *powatawi*. By contrast, *tuuhota* means to hurt or injure and *tuumoki* is to dream or die. In effect, *powa* emphasizes the opposition between the priestly healer and the witch, while *tuu* seems to place the individual shaman in an ambiguous relationship with death and illness.

The ceremonial year is divided into halves symbolizing the duality of life and death. In July, after the summer solstice, the benevolent rain-bringing *katcinas* return to the underworld for the winter half of the year, which lasts until the winter solstice at the end of December. The winter months are considered dangerous (*kya*); witches are thought to be especially active at this time, and people curtail their nighttime activities severely. The most dangerous month, December, is called *kyamüye*. But, in February the land is purified and made ready for planting. The purification ceremony is called *powamu* and the month, *powamüye*. During the winter months, the only *katcina* to appear on earth is Masau, the god of death. And during this time the dead are thought to conduct their ceremonies in the underworld. The world of the dead is, in fact, the mirror opposite of that of the living. But if life and death are complementary, the boundary between them must be maintained by the ceremonial use of *powa*.

The other Pueblos—the Zunis, Keresans, and Tanoans—had shamans called "Bears." They were thought to be possessed by the spirit of the bear while in a trance, they were the most powerful of all healers, and only they could cure illness caused by witchcraft. Not only did they derive their power from the bear, but their souls also entered and possessed bears who could

then be made to do the shamans' bidding.[2] During curing ceremonies, the shamans impersonated bears and were thought to
transform themselves into bears when engaging witches in
mortal combat. The bear shaman societies of the Rio Grande
Keresan Pueblos were the most elaborate and powerful, and
it is thought that the complex spread from the Keresans to
the Zunis and Tanoans. Rio Grande Keresan shaman societies
wielded far more political power than did those of the Tewas,
western Keresans, or Zunis. Not only did they appoint the
governing officials of the Pueblo—the caciques, war chiefs,
and fiscales—but these appointments were often made from
among their own membership.

Although Pueblo shamanism is most often depicted as lacking vision quests, trance states, and the use of psychoactive
plants to induce them, there is evidence enough to demonstrate the contrary.[3] Despite this retention of shamanism, however, even the Keresan Bear societies were charged with the
task of bringing rain and guarding the entire community from
misfortune. Nor were the shamans called upon to cure all diseases. A number of Rio Grande Keresan "doctor" societies existed; they cured ailments caused by chance or by breach of
tabu. Snake doctors cured snake bites. The thunderbird doctors
treated lightning shock and set bones, whereas ant doctors
cured all illnesses caused by contacts with ants.

Although the Hopis appear to have been antagonistic to
shamanism, for a period of time they had two medicine societies thought to have been borrowed from the Zunis.[4] The
basic Hopi pattern, however, relegated the shaman to a status
that can almost be called marginal.

Pueblo creation myths reflect the settled agriculturalists'
need for order and predictability. Whereas the myths of the
hunters and gatherers consist of disconnected episodes, those
of the Pueblos are marked by a complex structure and a plot
line that integrates episodes. The evolution of life from the un-
differentiated forms of the "first times" to the complex specia-
tion of the present world is carefully spelled out, as are the
reasons for the progression from one stage to the next. The cos-
mos is ordered into a series of lower "worlds" or stages of development of which the present is merely the most recent. The

consistent goal of each set of actions is the creation of a perfect order in which all the parts are harmoniously interrelated. The action which precipitates the flight from one world to the next is the destruction of that order either by witches or by imperfectly created beings.

In these myths, Coyote plays a far less important role than he or other trickster figures do in the myths of hunters and gatherers. Chaos and unpredictability are given far less leeway, and the creative aspects of Coyote are sharply separated from his "evil" actions. Many of the more archaic Coyote themes are retained, but they are most often placed in less pivotal positions. Coyote brings fire, but, instead of doing it of his own accord, the Keresans cast him in the role of a well-mannered messenger who brings the fire that has been wrapped in his tail by the underground creator Mother (Parsons 1974:194, 211). For all the Pueblos he is a guard warning of enemies, sighting game, and, at Taos, forecasting the weather (Parsons 1974:194). At Zuni, where the hunt animals are given special importance, Coyote is the hunt god of the west and the hunt society is named after him (Parsons 1974:188). But he is expunged entirely from themes of sexual conflict such as the conquest of the *vagina dentata* which, in the Hopi version, is accomplished by a medicine society (Stephen 1929:28). Although still associated with witchcraft and death, he seems not to be the major symbol of either in any of the Pueblos and he is not associated with any of the shaman societies. Nor is the coyote avoided but may be hunted and even eaten when game is scarce at Hopi and Jemez (Stephen 1929:22).

The ideal Pueblo individual is one who places the good of the community above his own desires. In order to achieve this, self-discipline and a sense of responsibility are assiduously cultivated. Disease is caused most often by breach of tabu or made likely by the individual's own bad thoughts. The Dionysian qualities so valued by the hunter are feared and tightly controlled by the Pueblo farmer. Control of supernatural power by individuals and dissociative states are disvalued, and great effort is expended to guarantee the orderly and predictable repetition of the agricultural cycle. Some anthropologists, inferring personality from values, world view, and social institutions, have represented the Hopis as repressed and have emphasized the conflict between the desires of the individual and the demands of the community without having a recourse to an earlier shamanistic tradition (Bennett 1946).

Navajo Adaptations

We have seen that, after their arrival in the Southwest, the Navajos made the transition from a major reliance on hunting to a subsistence economy based primarily on farming to which pastoralism was later added. During the seventeenth and eighteenth centuries their population increased and spread over a large area in western New Mexico and central and eastern Arizona. Throughout almost all of this territory, farming was marginal and pastoral pursuits came to dominate. As the population dispersed, the pueblitos that were formed during the period of intense Pueblo contact were abandoned. Low population density and transhumance precluded the development of community-wide ceremonials which marked the Pueblo agricultural cycle and curing societies. In consequence, Navajo ceremonies are almost exclusively healing rituals performed for individuals. In most other respects, however, the Navajos patterned their religion after that of the Pueblos.

Navajo curing ceremonies are referred to as "sings" (hatal), or "chants," and the ceremonialists who perform them as "singers" (hatałi). Like Pueblo priests, singers gain their knowledge of one or several ceremonies over long years of apprenticeship. The singer cures but does not diagnose the illness; diagnosis is done by "listening," "stargazing," or "hand trembling." Listeners and stargazers are rare, are always men, and have learned the procedures. By far the most common method of diagnosis is hand trembling, which is practiced by both men and women although, in our experience, women outnumber men as hand tremblers.

Hand trembling is said to be an unsought gift signaled by the shaking of the right arm. The person so chosen is thought to be possessed by the spirit of the supernatural Gila Monster. A ceremony must then be performed to control the involuntary shaking so that it does not become a disease and, at the same time, to introduce the individual to the status of diagnostician (Wyman 1936a). The hand trembler is a shaman because he is thought to be possessed while in a trance, although this method of diagnosis and the Hand-Tremblingway ceremony were borrowed after 1860 from the Apaches (Wyman and Kluckhohn 1938:28–29). All diagnosticians, however, are said to be in a trance state while practicing their art, and the origin of the stargazing rite mentions that it was caused by Coyote possession (Wyman 1936b).

Breach of tabu and witchcraft are the most frequently mentioned causes of disease. "Witchery" is the primary form of Navajo witchcraft and, as in the Hopi creation myth, its origin is attributed to First Man. Witches are associated with death and sibling incest, two of the most dangerous etiologic agents. To become a witch, an individual must also kill a close relative, preferably a sibling. In the myths of many sings, however, witches live in incestuous unions with their daughters. Some informants claim that the witch initiate must also eat part of the murdered relative's body. The effective means of working witchery is to touch the victim with a powder made of corpse flesh, thus bringing him into contact with a disease-causing object. Witches transform themselves into wolves, coyotes, dogs, or, less frequently, any of several other animals so that they may travel undetected. Witchery mirrors and is the evil opposite of Navajo religion. Not only is it based on the two great "dangers," incest and death, but witches band together and perform their own ceremonials using chants, sand paintings, body painting, and masks. Informants describe the proceedings as "just like a bad sing" (Kluckhohn 1962:34–35). As corpse powder is brought into contact with the victim, the illness is really "ghost sickness," and witchery is more properly thought of as a vector than as a cause of disease.

"Sorcery" is closely associated with witchery, and sorcerers participate in the witchery ceremonials. Sorcerers use spells to work their evil. The sorcerer must have a bit of the victim's personal excreta—such as hair, nails, feces—over which he casts his spell. Here, too, breach of tabu is the proximate cause of illness, as the excreta are buried by a grave or by a tree that has been struck by lightning, both considered "dangerous."

"Frenzy witchcraft" is primarily love magic, although it is also used in hunting, trading, and gambling. The master of this form of witchcraft uses a concoction made from datura and other plants in much the same way as "corpse powder" is used in witchery. Datura contains scopolamine and hyoscyamine and produces hallucinations, dissociative reactions, and, in large doses, coma. According to Navajo belief, the victim has only to touch the concoction for its effect to be felt. The purpose is to make the victim lose her senses and run away from her home in a sexual frenzy so that the witch may seduce her. Similarly, game animals fall easy prey to the hunter, and gamblers wager recklessly when witched in this manner.

An intrusive object may be injected into the body by a special form of witchcraft that has been translated as "wizardry" (Kluckhohn 1962:27). Most often, Pueblo, Ute, and Apache curers are consulted, and many Navajos believe that wizardry was borrowed from the Pueblos. Suckingway, the Navajo ceremonial cure, is thought to have been borrowed from the Chiricahua Apaches about a century ago (Haile 1950:296–97).

Most often, a tabu is breached by coming into contact with a dangerous object. There are literally hundreds of animals and natural phenomena thought to be dangerous in greater or lesser degree. Navajos recognize four classes of dangerous objects: animals, natural phenomena, healing ceremonies, and evil spirits (Wyman and Kluckhohn 1938). The most frequently mentioned animals are the bear, coyote, porcupine, snake, eagle, moth, ant, long-horned grasshopper, and camel cricket. Of natural phenomena, lightning and whirlwinds are the most common causes of disease, although water, hail, and the earth itself are sometimes mentioned.

Any ceremonial can cause illness. All powerful forces are dangerous, so that, when the Holy People are present during a ceremony, an individual may be affected. People who become ill in this way are thought to have the same illness that the ceremonial is said to cure. Transgressions of ceremonial tabus, such as that prohibiting cohabitation during a ceremony and for four days afterward, may cause illness. Breach of tabu by a couple during the mother's pregnancy can cause the child to be sick. A common statement is "my mother looked at a sand painting she was not supposed to see."

Contact with ghosts is one of the most common causes of illness. Any contact with a corpse, the dwelling where a death has occurred, Pueblo ruins, and even old artifacts will cause ghost sickness. A variety of mythical monsters are also included in the class of evil spirits, but diagnoses involving them are rare at present.

The principles of sympathetic magic, especially contagious magic, and the nature of supernatural power explain why many of these phenomena are thought to cause disease. Camel crickets and long-horned grasshoppers are associated with ghosts because they gather around dead bodies, for example. A sand painting is dangerous because it "attracts" supernatural power into the ceremonial arena for curing purposes, and those who are not protected (i.e., women) are at risk if they come into contact with it. Naturalistic explanations also account for why destructive whirlwinds and lightning are included as disease-causing agents. Many other etiologic factors, however, can only be understood in terms of the myths that account for each of the healing ceremonies. The association of butterflies and moths with incest is only one example. Despite the adequacy of some naturalistic explanations, a full appreciation of the coherence of the system depends on an understanding of the myths.

Navajos never attribute their illnesses to soul loss despite the importance of the soul, or wind (niłch'i), concept. At death the soul leaves the body and proceeds to the afterworld. Fainting and suffocation are signs of its departure and signal the final stages of an illness. A child's first laugh indicates that the soul has become attached to the body. Before this, death comes easily. Again during old age, the soul is loosely attached and death at this time is considered natural. The ghosts of infants and the aged are not thought to be so dangerous as those of people who die in the prime of life. Fainting is often attributed to contact with a ghost. It is contact that is mentioned, however, and not soul loss. Shock or fright resulting from contact with a ghost is known but rarely mentioned.

Belief in possession must be inferred from references to it in the myths. When patients are diagnosed, they are told either that they have been witched or that they have breached a tabu—that is, inadvertently come into contact with a dangerous object. Yet, when we read the recorded origin myths of the healing ceremonies or talk with ceremonialists, we find the principal diseases described in terms of possession. The myth of the stargazing ritual, for example, tells of the hero who was cured when he spat out Coyote's blood. Although an individual is most likely to get moth sickness by coming into contact with a moth, descriptions of the Mothway ceremony say that the patient will spit out moths that have lodged themselves behind his eyes. And the myth of Evilway tells how Coyote sent his ghost into the hero to witch him.

Navajos classify diseases by cause rather than by symptom, and each healing ceremony is known by the causal factor it is thought to counteract. Thus, Shootingway deals with illnesses caused by lightning, and Windway with wind-caused illnesses. Over seventy-five ceremonies have been identified. Their interrelationships and classification have occupied an important place in studies of Navajo religion. Ceremonies are grouped according to whether they are aimed at exorcising disease or protecting against infection and, beyond this, according to a variety of ritual procedures which set a given group of ceremonies off from others.

The concept of Beauty (hózhǫ́ǫ́) is opposed to that of Evil (hóchǫ́ǫ́). On the Beauty side are a group of rites known as Blessingways (hózhǫ́ǫ́jikehgo). These are short, lasting only two nights, and used to maintain harmony, to avert misfortune, and to bless all possessions and daily activities. The rites are used to consecrate ceremonial paraphernalia, to bless houses and flocks, and to aid in childbirth. The girls' puberty ritual and the wedding ceremony are largely comprised of Blessingway rites, and at least one Blessingway song must be included in every curing ceremony to protect against the effects of possible mistakes. Blessingway is used for prevention and protection rather than for cure. Although an individual "patient" is treated, Blessingway rites are thought to benefit the social group the patient represents. Unlike the paraphernalia of the curing sings, the mountain soil bundle of the Blessingway may be owned by the kin group, probably the coresident matrilineage (Wyman 1970:22). Thus, the Blessingways come closest to replicating the Pueblo communal ceremonies. Blessingway is also especially concerned with the uses of pollen and the creation and care of corn. As the ceremonies of the Pueblo agricultural cycle are intended to promote life through fertility and group well-being, so Blessingway lays special emphasis on life-giving supernatural power in all its forms, on the happiness of long life, the home, and the creation of living things.

Closely related to the Blessingways is the Lifeway group ('iinájikehgo), also of two nights' duration, the rituals of which are used for injuries due to accidents and for stubborn, chronic ailments. When used for the latter, they are performed in conjunction with a ritual from the sing normally used to cure the disease in question.

The Holyway ceremonials (diyinkehgo) comprise the largest of all the ceremonial groups. In addition to the familiar two- and five-night forms, several nine-night sings with public performances and masked dancers are included in this group. Although exorcistic in intent, Holyway ceremonials are "dominated by a pattern of behavior, theoretically directed by the Holy People, which concerns itself with the attraction of good and restoration of the patient" (Wyman 1975:16). In this regard Holyway ceremonials give the appearance of being incorporated into the conceptual framework of Blessingway rather than standing in opposition to the notion that hózhǫ́ǫ́ in and of itself has curative powers. In theory, the diseases cured by these sings result from trespass or offense against the gods, who then provide the cure. The emphasis on the Holy People and breach of tabu is reminiscent of the Hopi ceremonial societies which cure the disease caused by trespass against that domain of power they are thought to control. The Holy People are the masked gods of the Navajos and, like Pueblo katcinas, are impersonated in several of the sings. The Navajos consider the sings of the Holy People subgroup, especially Nightway, to have been derived from the Pueblos (Kluckhohn 1962:74).

Farthest removed from the Blessingways are the sings of the
Evilway group (hóchǫ́ǫ́jikehgo). The Evilways are design to
exorcise ghosts and thus cure sickness caused by them. And,
because witchery works its evil by bringing the victim into
contact with a powder made from a corpse, they are also
thought to counteract the bad effects of witchcraft. These ceremonies generally last for five nights and are more complex
than Blessingway rites. The myths of the major ceremonial,
Upward-reachingway, or Moving-upway (hanehnéhee), is the
only one that starts with the first creation and recounts the
entire story of the emergence from the underworlds. Many of
the Holyway sings have their Evilway "sides," and all healing
ceremonies must include at least one Blessingway song so that,
in terms of ceremonial practice at least, there is some integration of the blessing and exorcising aspects.

War and hunt ceremonies are no longer practiced and are, in
consequence, poorly recorded. Where they fit in the overall
classificatory scheme is not known.[5] Although the Blessingways and the Lifeways may be performed at any time of the
year, the exorcistic sings may be performed only during the
winter months.[6] The Enemyway, performed in the summer, is
the only exception. It is likely that this sing is a descendant of
the war purification rituals. Today, one of its major functions is
social. The evening dances serve the purpose of a coming-out
dance where potential mates meet. Most singers do not consider the Enemyway to be a real sing because it does not involve
the use of a rattle as the others do. We suspect that sometime
after the shift to pastoralism and the dispersal of the population, the Enemyway was modified so that it could serve this
increasingly important social function.

Blessingway is regarded by most Navajos as the backbone of
their religion. According to Wyman, it controls all the ceremonials and is an integrating force in Navajo culture (Wyman
1975:7). Singers of Blessingway believe that it developed before
all other ceremonies (Mitchell 1978:227; Wyman 1970:5). On
the other hand, singers of Evilway and some other, equally dangerous, ceremonies, are convinced that Evilway is the oldest
of Navajo ceremonies (Luckert 1981:xi; Franciscan Fathers
1910:362; Wyman and Bailey 1943:6).[7] Although the history of

Navajo ceremonialism cannot be reconstructed with any confidence, the question is of more than passing interest because it highlights the conceptual opposition that exists between *hózhǫ́ǫ́* and *hóchǫ́ǫ́*.

The Navajo creation myth is most similar to that of the Hopis. The emergence from a series of underworlds, each assigned a color and each ended by a natural catastrophe that forced the survivors to enter the next stage of existence, is replicated in the Navajo myth. Hopi worlds are brought to an end by the evil deeds of the people in general and especially of the witches, who never seem to be left behind. The Navajo account pays more attention to sexual antagonisms and sexual deviation than does the Hopi, however. Throughout the Navajo account, Coyote is the embodiment of evil. Karl Luckert in his book *Coyoteway* sees the Navajo Coyote as a "defamed hunter god" who was once a creator trickster but who, after hunting was abandoned, became the symbol of all that was evil and undesirable (Luckert 1979:3–12). Whereas the Pueblos made Coyote the servant of First Man or other creator gods, emphasize some of his more socially constructive characteristics, and attribute many of his sexual exploits to humans, the Navajos continue to assign Coyote a principal role in creation, witchcraft, and sexual deviance. Some versions of the Navajo creation myth say that Coyote was created even before First Man (O'Bryan 1956; Fishler 1953). An Evilway singer once told us that Coyote was *the* creator and that, although most Navajos did not know this, all of creation rested on his shoulders. In sum, the image of Coyote in Navajo myth is very much that of the shamanistic trickster creator at the same time he symbolizes all that is opposed to the concept of *hozhǫ́ǫ́*.

The Navajos, like the Pueblos, have polarized the concept of supernatural power and have made a corresponding twofold division in the ceremonial structure. Like the Hopis, they have emphasized breach of tabu without, however, stressing individual responsibility to the same degree. And both Navajos and Hopis, in contrast to the other Pueblos, appear to have abandoned belief in possession and soul loss. Indeed, we have seen that shamanism can hardly be said to be absent from Pueblo religion. Rather, all the Pueblos, except the Hopis, make sha-

manistic curing an important feature of their religious practices. In this regard also, the Navajos are more like the Hopis in
their antipathy to shamanistic practices, believing, correctly or
not, that hand-trembling, wizardry, and the sucking cure are all
of recent origin.

CHAPTER 3

Beliefs About Seizures

Although the identification of moth madness, frenzy witchcraft, and hand trembling with three recognizable types of seizures is relatively straightforward, it tells us little about where seizure disorders fit in the larger scheme of Navajo disease classification. Are these three etiologies, for example, subclasses of a larger category of aberrant behaviors, and, if so, is Coyote thought to be the primary etiological agent, the symbol of the irrational? This chapter examines how Navajos talk about seizures, how the myths explain them, and how Navajo beliefs differ from those of their Pueblo and Apache neighbors.

The Language of Spells

Navajos use different terms to refer to their illnesses depending on whether they have already been diagnosed, are seeking medical treatment, or are responding to specific questions concerning their symptoms posed by relatives or physicians. There is no need to identify symptoms during the course of diagnosis and treatment because the purpose of these activities is to discover and remove supernatural causes by magical means. The average Navajo is not conditioned to discourse about seizures with physicians or when asked to speak about disease in general. This is not, however, the case when family members must care for a patient. In this context Navajos describe their symptoms and pain accurately and in great detail (Landar 1967).

We were repeatedly impressed by the accuracy of the descriptions of seizures given by the patients and their families. Some purely descriptive terms are trembling (dits'gis), shaking (ditłid and the stem—ghał), and falling (−goh). Patients described loss of consciousness during a seizure as "my mind disappeared" (shini' 'asdiid) or "I was unconscious" (doo shił ééhózinda). Sometimes the sensation of something actually covering the mind or head was described as "being covered from above" (yaniłts'i). The sensation of spinning or twirling was often described as, "with me it turns around again" (shił nááhoomas) or "dizzy" (hodighááh). All of these terms were used freely by patients and their families when describing seizures to us because they indicated neither the circumstances which precipitated the episode nor its cause.

Somewhat removed from pure description are terms used by informants when talking about seizure disorders in general but rarely by patients talking about themselves. The verb stem tsaał refers to comas, faints, unconsciousness, and dying; it implies an underlying state of fear. The verb tłił is used where the ultimate state of dying is not implied; it is usually translated as stun. Like the Pueblos, Navajos use these terms to refer to the state of fear and shock experienced by those who come into contact with a ghost. Fear is the proximate cause but, except for ghosts, other dangerous beings are not usually identified. Seizures are not necessarily implied by these two terms, but they are often used in general discussions—leaving the listener to decide whether seizures are present or not.

There are, however, words denoting precipitating events or prior conditions which always imply the presence of convulsions. Diitła denotes an episode which occurs during a ceremony. When this happens, the afflicted individual is thought to be affected by the etiologic agent the ceremony is supposed to remove. It is not necessary for him actually to have had convulsions. Nevertheless, the term suggests the presence of a convulsive disorder, because if the condition is not treated it will ultimately lead to the convulsions of the grand mal seizure.

Still another word connoting convulsions is diigis, generally translated as "crazy," but most often used in reference to mental retardation, slowness, and ineptitude. Epileptics whose seizures begin early in childhood are also called diigis. Many informants said that the word is used only when the condition is chronic and has persisted since childhood. All agreed that it brought convulsions to mind and, as diigis is derived from the stem–gis, which means to turn or twist, we feel that it is correct to include it with terms used for seizures. Nevertheless, the vast majority of retarded children who are called *diigis* have never experienced seizures. Most often, when a chronic disorder of childhood is involved, breach of a tabu by one or both parents is suggested.

The terms denoting specific causes are those we have translated as moth madness, frenzy witchcraft, and hand trembling. *'Iich'ǫh* literally means falling into the fire and is the word for moth (*'iich'ǫhi*, one who falls into the fire). It is used to denote convulsions only in the event a diagnosis of moth madness has been made or incest is known to have taken place. A closely related word, *iich'ah*, means glans penis, considered dangerous and always covered when in the sweat bath.

Ajił'ee (frenzy witchcraft) is derived from the verb stem *jił*, to be lustful. Its use is restricted to episodes known to be caused by love magic. *Jił* refers only to the sexual excesses of women and to those few cases of men witched to make them lose in gambling. The condition caused by this type of witchcraft typically resembles a dissociative state and some complex partial seizures.

Ndishniih, to tremble or move the hand about (for the purpose of diagnosing), does not connote a state of wildness or excess despite the fact that the trembling is always thought to be involuntary, may vary from a fine tremor of the hand to rather violent motions of the whole arm, and can become uncontrollable. It is only used to refer to the behavior displayed by diagnosticians and caused by possession by Gila Monster.

The thematic prefix *tsi* connotes extreme behavior of all sorts, including drunkenness, violence, trembling, convulsions, and all irrational behavior. Literally, *tsi* means the manner in which one walks "in every direction"—that is, aimlessly and chaotically (Young and Morgan 1980:470). Yet lack of direction is equated with going to extremes, a natural consequence when constraints and direction are lacking. It is applied broadly and encompasses many behaviors. "Walking in all directions" (*tsi'naaghá*) connotes drunkenness and dizzyness. *Asdzáni yee tsi'naaghá* refers to sexual excess, going to extremes with women. *Tsi'ndidá* and *tsi'déyá* refer to any extreme act, a state of wild emotions, or a drunken state. *Tsi'ndiis'á* (caused them to go wild) is used in the myth of Mothway to describe the behavior of the Butterfly People after they committed sibling incest.

In daily speech Navajos most often use the terms descriptively without connoting a cause. In our opinion, however, *tsi* serves as the label for a major class of disorders. A ceremonialist who knew but did not perform Mothway and Frenzy-witchcraftway emphatically insisted that all conditions referred to by words with the *tsi* prefix imply generalized convulsions caused by incest. Regardless of the proximate cause, whether witchcraft, contact with a moth, or alcoholic intoxication, the condition will lead to convulsions and ultimately to incest itself if not cured. In effect, the causal arrow does not point in one direction only. Incest ultimately leads to seizures because one is in a state of wildness (*tsi*), but the sequence may also work in reverse; a person who is drunk or witched may become so "wild" that all rational controls are set aside so that incest is a likely outcome. According to this informant, all *tsi* behaviors are characteristic of Coyote, and all other referents to seizures are subsumed under *tsi* terms. Thus, because the Butterflies went wild and flew aimlessly, the use of *'iich'ąh* (moth sickness) is equated with the *tsi* state. *Ajiłee* is a subclass of *tsi* behavior. *Ndishniih*, however, is never said to be *tsi* even when the shaking is out of control.

Only the strictly descriptive terms do not connote supernaturally caused convulsions. Yet the description of signs and symptoms occurs only in a very restricted context, so that most discourse implies etiologic factors even in the absence of actual seizures. This was brought home forcibly when, in our attempt to identify epileptics in a community survey, we confined ourselves to using descriptive terms only. Singers and knowledgeable informants were asked who, in their community, was known to shake, fall to the ground, and lose consciousness. Known epileptics were, in fact, identified by this method. So too, however, were some completely asymptomatic individuals and people with a variety of conditions that did not involve seizures.

One young man responded to our questions by saying that he had a seizure disorder. When asked to describe his seizures, however, he was equally positive in stating that he had never fallen and convulsed. We asked him what made him think he had this kind of problem, and his answer was simply that he had anxiety dreams and attacks which indicated that, if a ceremonial was not performed soon, he would ultimately develop the kinds of seizures we had described.

In the same community, a prominent ceremonialist told us of a man who had convulsions in the past but who was now "just paralysed. He can't walk well any more either." It turned out that this man was himself a Shootingway singer and the father of an epileptic child in the study. During our interview with him, he demonstrated obvious left-sided dysfunction, hyperreflexia, and equivocal left Babinski reflex. He was able to walk a bit but gave the impression of a broken man with shaken self-esteem.

According to his account, he was helping out at an Evilway ceremony when, an hour after cutting some prayer sticks, "a dangerous thing for a ceremonialist to do," he felt a sharp pain in his knee and found he could not use his leg at all. That night he awoke to find the left side of his body paralysed. We suspected that he may have cast an embolus to the left femoral artery. Although he had visited the hospital three years earlier for left Bell's palsy with marked left-leg lag, he did not consider the two similar episodes as parts of the same illness. He was an acute observer, described his symptoms accurately, and did not confuse them with convulsions. He clearly distinguished his daughter's symptoms from his own, noting that he did not fall and tremble as she did. Nevertheless, Parker translated his account of the episode as, "Then he got a kind of convulsion. They call it *diitła*." Both Parker and the informant insisted that *diitła* was best thought of as a convulsion. To illustrate the point, the informant related an incident which took place some twenty years earlier: "I was at an Enemyway. A woman right next to me was skinning sheep. Suddenly she cried out, fell down, foamed at the mouth, and shook all over—*diitła*, that's what they call it." Although the term is used because of the ceremonial context and does not mean that everyone who has some sort of attack while attending a ceremony has seizures, the example of a woman who did have a seizure was used to illustrate why *diitła* is thought of as a seizure disorder.

One middle-aged man identified in the community survey told us of the monthly occurrence of fainting spells over a period of six years during which he only fell down once. The episodes were always associated with exertion, and at times he saw lights "like little sparks." There was no history of rheumatic fever, and the episodes did not sound like minor epileptic seizures. We thought it likely that he suffered from syncopal attacks, perhaps due to a heart condition.

The informant included a variety of complaints as part of his spells. When he was tired, his legs felt stiff. In the past, he would get violent while drunk. These conditions, he believed, were the early signs of what was later to become the fainting attacks. He believed that his dreams about werewolves coming after him, and dreams about falling from high places aggravated his condition. These examples suggest that people with a wide variety of ailments may be grouped together regardless of their actual symptoms.

Navajo nurses and interpreters also tended to use the English word "spell" to refer to disorders that a physician would not consider to be seizures. A middle-aged woman in hospital with severe hypothyroidism and possible hypopituitarism was brought to our attention when Navajo nurses complained that one of the ward patients was suffering from spells. The patient had a long history of anemia, and her spells were described by hospital personnel as falling and blacking out. She was also seen just sitting and staring. At times she would have the urge to vomit but could only gag. On occasion she became frantic, so that side rails were attached to her bed. One of the nurses said that she would yell and run around the ward. Attending physicians had seen her in a comatose state. The patient left the hospital without permission and returned home, where she was diagnosed and treated for frenzy witchcraft. Neither she nor any member of the family had ever seen anyone with seizures. To them, the patient's symptoms were those typically exhibited by victims of love magic.

Another hospital patient, a married woman in her thirties,

complained of headache, sore throat, chest pain, lack of blood circulation, involuntary spasms of the neck muscles, dripping of saliva, and abdominal pain. The physical examination was negative, and her complaints disappeared after antidepressant medication was given. The diagnosis at the time was "psychoneurotic reaction with conversion and depression." She told us that when she said she suffered from spells she was referring primarily to the involuntary spasms of the neck muscles and the salivation. It was our impression that the involuntary nature of these spasms was the focus of concern. A year later, this patient was readmitted to hospital and committed to the state insane asylum with a diagnosis of catatonic schizophrenia.

Several schizophrenics were described by their families as being *tsi'ndidá*. As reported, their behaviors sounded very much like violent paranoia. After a period of observation, however, only one of these patients was diagnosed as a paranoid schizophrenic. The others suffered from other forms of schizophrenia. After careful questioning we discovered that none had actually exhibited the violent behavior attributed to them at the time they were brought to hospital.[1] The families, as well as some of the patients, were afraid that violent and "wild" states would result if some sort of treatment was not received immediately.

In sum, people with a wide variety of symptoms are grouped together if there is any evidence of irrational behavior of any sort or, in the absence of symptoms, if there is reason to believe that a disease process has begun which will ultimately lead to irrationality. Mental retardation, obsession, extremes of action or thought, intoxication, and unconsciousness indicate that the mind is not in full control and are identified by the more knowledgeable with the irrational excesses of Coyote. There are, however, some terms not in the *tsi* category that are used to suggest that possible presence of seizures. Navajos are reluctant to speak openly about incest and prefer to use ambiguous terms of reference. When *diigis* is used, for example, it is clear that the condition began in childhood and is therefore most probably the result of a parent's transgression which might be nothing more embarrassing than that the mother came too close to a sand painting. But, because incest might also have been involved, the speaker is able to talk about the child without making a direct accusation.

Myth Background

We have already seen that hand trembling was borrowed from the Apaches during the nineteenth century. The myth of Hand-tremblingway is short and poorly integrated into the larger corpus of Navajo myth. It features a supernatural, Gila Monster, who figures prominently in only one other healing ceremony, Flintway. The hand-trembling trance is the mark of the ritual's shamanistic origins, yet the shaking of the arm is not said to be tsi'ndidá; thus, this form of diagnosis must be considered as a separate phenomenon. Stargazing and listening, on the other hand, involve possession by Coyote and, although their myths of origin are not well known, they were probably thought to cause seizures or other tsi behaviors when not performed properly.

The Mothway origin story differs considerably from the usual pattern of Navajo ceremonial myths. There is no single hero who gains knowledge and power through his exploits. And punishment from transgression, usually emanating from supernatural sources, is here a self-destructive act representing the internal sanction of guilt resulting from incest (Spencer 1957:148–50). The story relates how the Butterfly People are led by a bisexual god, Begochidi, who was born at Riverward Knoll, the place where plants and butterflies originated and where the Sun fertilized both the male and female plants. Born of the Sun and the flowers, Begochidi in his turn fertilizes the male and female Butterflies so that they never need to marry aliens (Haile 1978). After Begochidi leaves for another country where there is game, the Butterfly People decide it is better to commit incest than to marry outsiders. This, however, makes them go wild and, like moths, rush into some fires that had been built nearby. Later, when the healing ceremony is performed, they were "out of their minds," staggering about any old way. Coyote alone had medicines for cases of incest, and these were used to cure the supernatural siblings, Dawn Boy and Dawn Girl, who had emulated the butterflies' behavior and had also become sick. Although convulsions are not described, present-day Navajos invariably regard the major epileptic seizures to be the condition referred to in the myth because epileptics, like moths, fall into fires.

Today Mothway is extinct; our knowledge of it comes from Haile's published account and from one of our informants, an elderly woman who had the ceremony performed for her in her youth. In the myth account, the ceremony is conducted by Bear Man. Only Coyote had medicine for countering the effects of incest. This medicine was made from the generative organs of male and female sibling coyotes, yellow and blue foxes, badgers, and bears. There were also four Moth medicines. These were herbs not identified in the account. The Moth medicines were boiled over a fire and then combined with the Coyote medicines. After this, the Fire Ceremony was performed. A kilt of coyote skin was wrapped around each of the patients (Dawn Boy and Dawn Girl), after which they drank the medicine concoction. Finally, with their buttocks touching one another, they vomited the moths that were inside them, and these in turn were thrown into the fire.

Our informant had committed incest with an older brother around the turn of the century, when she was about twenty years old. The relationship was discovered when she had a fainting spell during which she lost consciousness and fell into the fire. Quite likely this was an hysterical anxiety attack, although the scars on her arm attested to the fact that she had done injury to herself.

Her account of the five-night ceremonial differed in some details from the version recorded by Haile. The Coyote medicines were made from the semen and vaginal discharges of a sibling set of coyotes rather than the genitalia of all the related animals. "A white curtain was put up inside the ceremonial hogan and around both patients. Within this curtain the patients had sexual intercourse as part of the curing ritual. Both wore fox skins representing their tail similar to a Nightway dancer. While the patients were copulating, they howled like whirling coyotes. When intercourse was over, the singer caught some of the semen of both patients which was then applied to the prayer stick prepared for an offering."[2] Finally, they were bidden to drink the Coyote and Moth medicines and then to face away from each other while inducing vomiting. There were no further episodes of fainting, and the patient was able to marry and lead a normal life thereafter. Nevertheless, recalling this painful and traumatic episode in her life provoked weeping throughout the interview.

The story of Frenzy-witchcraftway follows the adventures of a human hero who is given love and game magic by the gods (Spencer 1957:134–48; Kluckhohn 1962:36–42, 158–74, 177–88). The principal events are flirtation with and ridicule by Hopi women; a ceremony of gods conferring powers of love and game magic; marriage to Hopi maidens; seduction of Hopi virgins while disguised as a butterfly; theft of the hero's wives by the supernatural White Butterfly; the hero's retaliation for this by overcoming and killing him in a contest.[3]

The hero accomplishes the seduction by transforming himself into a butterfly which flutters into the girls' chamber and attracts their notice by its beauty. The sisters attempt to capture the butterfly in order to copy its pattern in their weaving and are thus enticed from their chamber into the light of day. Although aware they are doing wrong, they are unable to resist.

In the hero's absence, White Butterfly seduces and abducts his wives. The scene is not described, but the evidence of seduction is the tracks followed by the hero in his pursuit. Informants maintain that White Butterfly had the same kind of love magic as the hero's. After a contest of strength and wits, the hero kills White Butterfly with a blow to his head. As the head splits open, a host of butterflies flies up in a cloud. At the very end of the story, the hero sees to it that the "moths" that emerged from White Butterfly's head come back from the sky in the form of rain.

In the version recorded by Haile, there is a duplication of the seduction of the hero's wives by White Butterfly, in which Coyote appears to the women disguised as the hero. The hero, meanwhile, has been left to wander senseless in Coyote's form.

He is restored to his former shape by peeling off Coyote's skin as he is passed through several hoops. This episode is essentially the same as that found in Evilway.

In the myth no mention is made of teaching this ceremony to humans. Frenzy-witchcraftway is used to cure the effects of the use of love or game magic by witches. All informants stress the point that no one learns the ritual by itself because then it is nothing but evil and very dangerous. Instead, it must be learned in conjunction with Blessingway to protect the singer. And some say that if a man learns Blessingway first he never bothers to learn Frenzy-witchcraftway.

The victim of frenzy witchcraft is believed to lose her mind and to go into a state of lustful frenzy. Women so witched will go crazy, tear off their clothes, and go after the man who has witched them. A distinguishing feature of the ritual is the ingestion of datura by the patient, a procedure which recreates a state of "mindlessness" which may then be cured in a ritually controlled setting.

Pueblo Associations

The association of the butterfly and a bisexual fertility god with incest and seduction is derived from Pueblo, especially Zuni and Keresan, myths. *Awonawilona*, the creator god of the Zunis, is a "He-She," bisexual, life-giving power (Stevenson 1904:22). His first act of creation is to turn himself into the sun. Subsequently, he impregnates a human who gives birth to a son called *Paiyatemu*. Earlier, while the first humans are searching for the "Middle Place" where the Zunis are supposed to settle, a brother and sister are sent to help with the search. They commit incest and give birth to children who are the prototypes of the *Koyemsi*, or Mudhead, clowns. The incest is done while the brother is "crazed for love" (Stevenson 1904:22; Cushing 1896:32). Thereafter, the pair become hideously ugly with great knobs on their heads. Ten children are born of this union. The firstborn is a hermaphrodite with the form of a woman but the stature and strength of a man. "From the mingling of too much seed in one kind comes the 'two-fold one kind' 'hlamon, man and woman combined." The other children are remarkably ugly and malformed, without sense and, although male in appearance, without sex.

Paiyatemu is an archetypal trickster. He is always surrounded by butterflies, playing his seductive flute from which the butterflies emerge as objectified musical notes. In reality, he is the sacred butterfly—as the story of his death and resurrection makes plain (Tyler 1964:147–49, 197). Paiyatemu's evil sisters kill him and hide his heart and head. The oldest sister, who has stolen his flute, blows into it and from it come the butterflies of the directional colors. The last is multicolored and is Paiyatemu himself. What then follows is the story of the seduction of the Pueblo maidens as it appears in Frenzy-witchcraftway. Presumably, this is also an act of sibling incest, although the myth does not make a point of this. Paiyatemu in the form of a butterfly enters the room where the evil sisters are weaving baskets. Wishing to copy the designs on his wings, they pursue him, throwing various articles of their clothing in an attempt to net him, until they are all naked and fall asleep. Paiyatemu then takes off his butterfly disguise and blows upon his flute, whereupon each of the evil maidens comes out as a crazily flying butterfly, flying without direction.

Paiyatemu is a handsome clown who bears the shield of the sun on his journey and at times entertains him by playing his flute. A foil of the sun, he is funny and senseless and is allowed to do as he pleases (Tyler 1964:142–43). He is also the fertilizing and sexual power of the sun. Born of a mortal woman and the sun, he uses music to seduce women, all the while surrounded by myriads of butterlies. At Sia and Acoma he is the Koshare clown patron; at Zuni he is the father of the Newekwe clowns, as well as the patron of the Koyemsi. In his "daylight mood and appearance," Paiyatemu is gross and funny, his jokes are "reversals," and he is thoughtless, loud, and uncouth. At the same time he is the god of dew, dawn, and fertility (Cushing 1896:439).

The bumps on the heads of the Koyemsi are filled with all kinds of seeds, and they possess the most potent love magic. The Koyemsi are the most dangerous of all kachinas. If anyone touches a Koyemsi while he has his paint on, that person will surely go mad. They carry the sacred butterfly in their drum to make people follow them, and anyone who does so will go crazy. The butterfly love charm affects everyone but especially young girls, who must go after anyone who has it (Bunzel 1932b:871–72, 947; Tyler 1964:198, 200).

Although Hopi parallels are less detailed, we still find the butterfly associated with a god of fertility. *Muingwu*, the spirit of germination who created all seeds and plants, sits on "Flower Mound" with all the sacred birds and butterflies before him. The Hopis refer to butterflies as the pets of *Muingwu* (Stephen 1969:333, 1252, 1254).

Navajos believe that Mothway and Frenzy-witchcraftway are closely related—in part, because they both originate at Riverward Knoll, the hill where the fertilization of the medicinal plants occurs and where *Begochidi* is conceived. Despite the prominence of the butterfly symbol and sexual themes in both myths, however, Navajos associate these stories with Coyote and believe that the ceremonies are not only closely related to each other but also to Coyoteway and Mountaintopway.[4] Coyote medicines are used in Mothway. The Moth medicines are, quite likely, the same as those used in Frenzy-witchcraftway. A Coyote episode, duplicating one involving White Butterfly, is inserted into Frenzy-witchcraftway. Some Navajos even think of Mothway as the "Rabid Coyote branch of Coyoteway," although, in our experience, this ritual is used as a substitute for Mothway now that it is extinct (Kluckhohn 1962:230). In our view, Coyote is employed as the symbol of all that is evil in these ceremonies and integrates materials borrowed from the Pueblos during the eighteenth century into the larger Navajo structure which polarizes good and evil.

But if the major myth themes were borrowed from the Pueblos, the severity of the punishment for incest seems entirely Navajo. The Pueblos do not believe that seizures are caused by incest or any specific etiology. Zunis most often attribute seizures with an onset during childhood to the killing of a game animal by a parent who did not perform the proper hunt ritual. Today, this can most easily happen when a rabbit or deer is run down by an automobile. Tewas believe that when a child has seizures it is caused by an "evil" wind which, in turn, is most often thought to have been sent by a witch. The Hopis do not believe that any one cause of childhood seizures is more likely than another. Among all these groups, breach of tabu by one or both parents or witchcraft is assumed.

When seizures begin later in life (that is, after age sixteen or so), the Pueblos believe that the patient bears some responsibility for his affliction. Either some tabu has been breached or, especially among the Hopis, bad thoughts have made him susceptible to witchcraft. Sudden fright or shock is also thought to precipitate seizures among adults. Zunis spoke about seeing a deceased spouse at, or soon after, a funeral. Hopis thought the shock of hearing about a loved one's demise was also a cause. Tewa informants mentioned witchcraft more than anything else, and frequently said that a witch would cause a bad wind to enter the victim. None of the Pueblos thought that any of the causes mentioned resulted in seizures more often than other untoward results.

Sibling incest, we have seen, is thought by the Zunis to create hermaphrodite and asexual children. In the past if not today, the Zunis thought that clan incest would cause an earthquake which would release wild animals from underground (Parsons 1974:53). Neither familial nor clan incest were thought by the Hopis to do any harm to the participants and, when asked why one should not enter into such relationships, the average Hopi could give no specific reason beyond "they are of the same blood"; when pressed on the subject, they "appeared baffled and could not understand how one could seriously raise the point." Some thought that clan incest might be punished after death, but no specific retribution was mentioned (Brandt 1954:165, 206–10). Tewa informants felt that there was no punishment for incest, either social or supernatural, other than the bad reputation the family would have.

Although none of our Pueblo informants spoke of love magic, an episode observed by Stevenson shows that the "crazy" behavior caused by Zuni love magic also included seizure-like activity (Stevenson 1904:398–402). It seems that a handsome youth about seventeen years old took a twelve-year-old girl by the hands and asked her to go with him. According to the girl, she began to "tremble" as soon as she was touched. By her parents' account, she was "crazy" a short time after she got home. By the time Stevenson arrived on the scene, the boy had confessed to using a "love philtre" and the girl was on the floor, "every member of her body in violent motion. When asked to tell her story, the spasms made it almost impossible for her to articulate, and her head was not still for an instant." Later, the boy claimed he could remove the spell, but when he again touched the girl, "she was almost thrown into convulsions by the touch." Stevenson believed she had seen a severe case of hysteria, and we are inclined to agree.

The youth described how, on a visit to the Keresan Pueblo of Santo Domingo, he had learned the technique from one of the members of a healing society and how he and his friend had cast a spell on two girls of the village. Once touched with the "root medicine," the girls went to their home where they soon "felt their hearts flying around. Each girl sat still a minute, then jumped up and turned around like a top, then slept a moment, and then threw her arms wildly about. They could not keep their heads or their legs still. They jumped up and ran about the streets. We did not make these girls our wives. They were too crazy. In a short time they died." This story shows that seizures were among the effects of love magic, although none of our Pueblo patients or informants ever mentioned love magic as the cause of seizures.

Apache Associations

The Apaches treated incest as a civil crime and did not believe that it caused either seizures or any other illness. There was no ceremony against it or its aftereffects, and the offenders' kinsmen were in no way tainted by it (Goodwin 1969:309, 416–24, 427; Opler 1965:59–61, 249–51). Coyote committed the first act of incest when he seduced his daughter. Incest was viewed with horror, and the offenders were thought to be witches. If discovered in the act, a kinsman could kill them on the spot. Otherwise they were brought before the chiefs for trial. Most often the man was thought to be the witch and the woman his victim. The woman was usually able to save herself by confessing that her partner was a witch. Offenders who were old enough to be witches were killed or banished. There was no distinction made between sibling and father-daughter incest except that siblings were often too young to have knowledge of witchcraft. In such cases, the boy was banished from the tribe. The girl, however, stayed with her parents because she had no other way to survive. Among the matrilineal Western Apaches, clan and phratry endogamy were also forbidden. If people of the same clan married and refused to divorce, it was thought they would give birth to deformed or insane children. The parents, however, only suffered ridicule. There was also the belief that incest offenders would not be able to have children by a later marriage.

The Apaches also had love magic which was, especially in the case of the Western Apaches, very similar to Navajo frenzy witchcraft. The Western Apaches believed, for example, that the source of love power was a hill with plants and butterflies (Goodwin 1969:304–9; Opler 1965:151–53). The Chiricahua also associated the butterfly with sexual desire but saw it as representing the flightiness of women generally. Love magic was also closely identified with hunt magic, as it was among the Navajos. The crucial difference lay in the fact that the Apaches did not believe that its practitioners were really witches or that the consequences were serious, although an "overdose" could cause insanity. Love magic was linked neither with Coyote nor with incest and, although its practitioners did not often boast openly of their powers, they were not averse to selling their services. Anyone, it appears, could learn enough to practice the magic himself.

Navajos who practiced frenzy witchcraft were distinct from witches, wizards, and sorcerers in that they did not participate in the "witches sabbath" and did not behave as were-animals. Nevertheless, the Navajos clearly thought that frenzy witchcraft was a malevolent activity as dangerous as other forms of witchcraft. The price of initiation was the killing of a sibling and, according to some of Kluckhohn's information, there was an association with sibling incest as well (Kluckhohn 1962:40–411, pp. 177, 179). We found no cases of love magic among the Pueblo epileptics and hysterics, and Keith Basso (1969) does not report any instances in his study of contemporary Western Apache witchcraft. This is in sharp contrast to the number of cases of frenzy witchcraft found today on the Navajo reservation.

Some Questions

This comparison of Navajo beliefs and myths with those of the Pueblos and Apaches raises some questions regarding when and for what purpose they were developed. The Navajos, we have seen, were part of a migration of Athabascan speakers who penetrated the Southwest sometime before the arrival of the Spaniards in the sixteenth century and who only gradually became distinguishable as separate tribes as they occupied different areas and developed different economies. The Western Apaches, like the Navajos, became agriculturalists and developed matrilineal descent and exogamous clans and clan groups. Their contacts with the Pueblos were less intense, however, and many Puebloan traits may even have been borrowed from the Navajos and not directly from the Pueblos. The eastern Apaches—Chiricahuas, Mescaleros, Jicarillas, and Lipans—although exposed to agriculture, continued to rely primarily on hunting and, like most North American hunting and gathering tribes, had bilateral descent. All of these tribes, however, had a preference for matrilocal residence after marriage. We assume that the Navajos' beliefs about incest were the same as those held by the other southern Athabascans—namely, they made no great distinction between father-daughter and sibling incest, believing that all forms of familial incest derived from Coyote. There was, by this analogy, no specific supernatural sanction beyond the idea that, because the offender was a witch, he might go out of his mind if he could not retain control over his supernatural power.

The Navajos developed the idea that the breach of the sibling incest tabu caused one of the most fearful of all illnesses and, in the process, borrowed Pueblo myths and symbols. Yet the Pueblos do not appear to have been overly concerned about incest, clan endogamy, or, in recent years at least, love magic.

Navajos think of the Mothway legend as an explanation of the prohibition against sibling and clan incest. There is no complementary belief about father-daughter incest. Why was it necessary to borrow a Pueblo myth, and why give salience to sibling and clan incest? Most anthropologists believe that the Navajos and Western Apaches only developed matrilineal descent and a clan system after they learned agriculture in the Southwest. The prohibition was, according to this view, given salience because the descent system was newly developed. But, as we have pointed out, the Navajos would already have prohibited sibling incest and, if a further strengthening of the tabu were necessary when it was expanded to include clan incest, we should expect the Western Apaches also to have emphasized sibling and clan incest.

A more plausible explanation is that the original intent was to encourage intermarriage with the diverse groups of Pueblos who joined the Navajos after the Pueblo Revolt. Mothway specifically mentions Hopi, and the primordial act of incest took place before White House pueblo in Canyon de Chelly on land which today belongs to people of the Coyote Pass clan, a clan said to be descended from Jemez Pueblo refugees. The Hopis are also known to have lived in the canyon during the eighteenth century (Hill 1936:3–4).

Incest was committed in an attempt to avoid marriage with foreign groups, not marriage with other Butterfly People. The Butterfly chiefs express a desire to retain community endogamy when they say "at the time you became pregnant with those children, no help came to you in any way from those places from which their marriage is now offered to you. . . . your daughter would be one place somewhere and your son would be another place, but you would be crying for them." This suggests that prior alliances and reciprocal relations with the other groups did not already exist (Haile 1978:187).

The Pueblos with whom the Navajos had the most intense contacts—Jemez, Hopi, the western Keresans, and Zuni—all had matrilineal, exogamous clans. Some of the larger "pueblitos," as well as the early Navajo populations in Canyon de Chelly, which included Hopis as well as Jemez, must have contained a very large number of exogamous descent groups.[5] Under such conditions, according to Kathleen Gough, "there would be a tendency to marry back into father's clan and so form small knots of closely in-marrying groups within the larger political unit, thus leaving the larger unit without a firm basis for structuring its relations as a whole" (Gough 1961: 651).[6] Certainly this tendency would have been very strong in settlements where people of different languages and cultures were thrown together. In order to prevent the fragmentation of such groups, marriage prohibitions developed which forced individuals to seek mates from clans not already allied by marriage in the present or immediately preceding generation.

If, as many believe, matrilineal descent developed only after the Navajos adopted agriculture, there might have been some need to emphasize the importance of the basic rule of clan exogamy.[7] But this development is most likely to have occurred during the century prior to 1690, when Navajos and large numbers of Pueblo refugees formed joint settlements over a period of eighty years. Prior to 1690, the Navajos and the Western Apaches would have had a preference for marriage into father's clan because this form of marriage permits small populations with limited resources to protect their holdings by cementing alliances with only one or two other descent groups.

Today neither the Navajos nor any of the matrilineal Pueblos permit marriage into the father's clan. Among the Navajos, marriage between individuals whose fathers are of the same clan is also prohibited. And, in earlier days, marriage into mother's father's and father's father's clans may also have been discouraged.[8] For all of these prohibitions to have been in force, there would have had to have been many more exogamous descent groups than are presently found among the Navajos or any of the Pueblos. This could only have occurred when Navajos and several Pueblo groups lived together in settlements that maintained contact with each other.

During the latter half of the eighteenth century, the Navajo population grew and the dispersed settlement pattern, which is so characteristic of the seminomadic pastoralist, came into being. We think that the myth of Mothway was reinterpreted at this time to express a concern with sibling and clan incest in-

stead of group endogamy because familial incest became more
of a problem when many families were isolated for much of the
year and because the need to maintain extensive marriage restrictions lessened. Some of our informants, however, insist
that marriage into father's clan also causes moth sickness;
thus, it is possible that some element of the prohibition against
endogamy persists to the present.

The efficacy of social controls is an important factor in determining the amount of attention paid to the problem of incest.
Pueblo communities were tightly structured and so densely
populated that the opportunities for clandestine acts stood little chance of going undetected. Supernatural sanctions may
have been less necessary, especially when we consider that the
Pueblos, especially the Hopis, had been matrilineal for many
centuries. The Western Apaches also lived in what Goodwin
has called "local groups" composed of several "family clusters"
(or extended families), which corresponded to the Navajo camp
(Goodwin 1969:123–92). These local groups had recognized
leaders who were formally chosen, installed, and instructed.
Families living apart from a family cluster were rare, as were
family clusters that were not part of a local group. Although
the Apaches were more mobile than the Pueblos, they rarely
did anything alone. People seldom traveled, hunted, or went
gathering alone not only because of enemies but also because
of possible accident and injury. Goodwin found mature men
who had never spent a night alone, and even the less sedentary
Chiricahuas had a special treatment for loneliness (Opler
1965:37, 429).

How different were the pastoral Navajos, who spent much of
the year in relative isolation in residence groups composed of
one extended family from which nuclear families might separate for a variety of purposes and for varying lengths of time.
Sheepherding is often a solitary occupation, and there is no
dearth of stories telling of chance encounters between travel-
ing men and single women who were tending sheep. The
chance of discovery, in our opinion, was far less for the Navajos
than for any of the Apaches, and the fear of community reaction correspondingly weaker. There would be under these conditions a greater need for supernatural sanctions.

This reconstruction is highly speculative. Although it accounts for some of the observations, it does not explain the position of father-daughter incest in Navajo culture or the importance of love magic in the Navajo witchcraft belief complex. More important, the argument is based solely on inference made from myths and general statements about social regulations. There is, for example, considerable emphasis placed on sexual deviance and sexual excess in the Navajo creation myths. The separation of the sexes in the third underworld is a pivotal episode that propels the survivors of the flood into the present. The cause for the separation is always presented as a conflict between the sexes and as an experiment in gender autonomy, the consequences of which are sexual aberrations and the birth of evil monsters. But whether this emphasis placed on sexual conflict and sexual practices, including incest and seduction by witchcraft, indicates that sexual antagonisms and anxiety are central to Navajo character cannot, in our opinion, be ascertained by myth analysis alone but must be confirmed by data obtained from living people.

Chapters 6 through 8 examine individual cases to see whether beliefs about incest actually influence the way epileptics are diagnosed and treated by their families either by suspecting them of having committed incest or of being victims of frenzy witchcraft. In effect we will look for the reflection of myth in contemporary Navajo social life.

CHAPTER 4

The Epidemiology

of Seizures and

Pseudoseizures

In this book and in common medical usage, "seizure" is a descriptive term applied to any instance of altered consciousness, convulsions, or brief episodes of altered behavior. From the beginning, however, the term "epilepsy" has been used to designate a group of patients who were thought to have more in common than just their symptoms. The word is Greek and means attacked, or seized. The Greeks believed that all epileptics suffered from one disease—namely, possession by the gods. Modern medicine's understanding of epilepsy may be said to have begun in the late nineteenth century with the investigations of Hughlings Jackson in England and Jean Martin Charcot in France. Jackson outlined a neurological theory of epilepsy, while Charcot separated epilepsy from hysteria more emphatically than any of his predecessors. Jackson's principles were publicly demonstrated by William Macewan who "was probably the first surgeon to localize the cerebral focus by inference from the motor or sensory signs" of the epileptic seizure (Temkin 1971:x, 385).

Etiologically it is misleading to think of epilepsy as one disease. There are many causes of this symptom cluster, just as there are for the symptom cluster of nausea and vomiting. A better term would be "the epilepsies." The epilepsies do, however, share certain physiological characteristics.[1] Clusters of neurons in some part of the brain begin to discharge impulses in a disorganized fashion. The parts of the body controlled by the affected neurons respond with disorganized activity such as convulsions or tremors, or by loss of normal function such as loss of consciousness, paralysis of a limb, or localized numbness. The condition is also chronic, marked by the repeated occurrence of seizures. By monitoring the brain with electrodes, an electroencephalographer can often detect abnormal brain waves, either localized in one part of the brain or coming from all parts at once.

Although epilepsy can begin at any age, the majority of patients have their first seizure before the age of twenty. In fact, the age of onset is often related to the cause. Perinatal injuries, severe hypoxia, developmental brain defects, and genetic metabolic defects are common causes of epilepsy among infants and the newborn. Brain infections such as meningitis and encephalitis often result in damage to some brain cells with a subsequent development of epilepsy. Many children experience seizures during periods of high fever caused by infection in parts of the body other than the brain. Only a very small percentage of these febrile seizures persist after the age of four, however. Head trauma is one of the most common causes of seizures among adults, although brain tumor must also be suspected, as about 40 percent of all patients with brain tumors have seizures. Later in life, seizures may be caused by cerebrovascular attacks.

Despite medicine's increased ability to determine the various causes of epilepsy, no known cause can be found or reasonably presumed for a large proportion of seizures. Until a very few years ago, genetic predisposition was thought to be the cause of what was called "idiopathic" epilepsy. Today most experts do not believe that heritability plays as large a role as the proportion of patients whose seizures have been diagnosed as idiopathic might suggest. That genetic factors are involved, however, is indicated by the fact that people with a family history of epilepsy have a higher incidence of seizures than the population in general. In addition, the electroencephalogram tracings of asymptomatic relatives of patients with some forms of epilepsy show a higher incidence of abnormal discharge than is found among the rest of the population.

Epilepsy involves recurrent seizures, so that an individual's first seizure does not, of itself, indicate the presence of epilepsy. Nervous system infections, metabolic imbalance, and transient reactions to a head injury may all result in a seizure episode without putting the individual at risk for further seizures. Among epileptics an almost infinite number of stimuli may trigger seizure activity. Fatigue, alcohol abuse, and infection, for example, commonly precipitate attacks in people whose epilepsy is otherwise well controlled. Despite the great variability in thresholds and types of seizures and in the unpredictability of its course during the patient's lifetime, some features appear with striking frequency and some attacks are remarkably similar for many people.

The growing emphasis on physiological mechanisms and electroclinical correlations has led to a classification of the epilepsies by the localization of the electrical abnormality in the brain. The major division is between generalized (centrencephalic) seizures, where the activity is spread over the entire cerebral cortex, and partial (focal) seizures, which occur when only one part of the brain is involved. Generalized seizures have bilateral motor activity and involve loss of consciousness. Loss of consciousness may or may not occur in partial seizures depending upon the part of the brain initially affected and the subsequent involvement of other brain structures. There is an approximate correspondence between the sites of the brain where electrical abnormality occurs and the clinical manifestation of the seizure.

Generalized Seizures

The term epilepsy began its career by designating the symptoms of the major, or *grand mal*, seizure, currently referred to as a *tonic-clonic seizure*. To this day, over 60 percent of all individuals diagnosed as epileptic have tonic-clonic seizures. A sudden burst of discharges involving the whole brain occurs without warning. The patient falls to the ground unconscious. Then, in the tonic phase, the patient goes rigid and often gives a short cry due to the contraction of the diaphragm and chest muscles. The eyes may roll up or turn to one side, and the tongue may be bitten. After this, a period of jerky, *clonic*, spasms alternately flex and extend the muscles of the head, face, and extremities. During this phase there may be injury to the self as well as incontinence. Cyanosis is generally marked. Breathing is deep, and there is sweating and salivation. Subsequent to the seizure, the patient may waken in a confused state (postictal twilight state) and even display some bizarre behavior. Sometimes patients may be hard to arouse, sleep for hours, and awaken with headache or sore muscles. Although most tonic-clonic seizures last for only a few minutes, some patients develop a series of seizures with no letup or a continuous, prolonged seizure. This is a serious condition known as *status epilepticus* which may lead to death if immediate care is not provided.

A variety of other generalized seizures have also been recognized. Sometimes patients only exhibit the tonic or the clonic aspects of the seizure. Between the ages of four and twelve, *absence seizures* often occur. These have been known as *petit mal* because they are of such brief duration, no more than a few seconds, that they often go unrecognized and untreated. During the brief lapse of consciousness, the child stares vacantly and neither speaks nor hears. Subsequently, activity is resumed with no period of stuporousness. Equally brief are *atonic seizures*, during which the child simply falls to the ground; *myoclonic seizures*, which are sudden, brief, and massive, involving either the entire body or confined to the extremities, face, or trunk; and *infantile spasms*, during which the child is jerked into a fetal position with the knees drawn up. Many children with infantile spasms are also mentally retarded.

Partial Seizures

All partial seizures begin in one part of the brain and, because different parts of the brain control different parts of the body as well as mental and sensory functions, their signs and symptoms are varied and often quite complex. Many patients exhibit behaviors easily mistaken as psychiatric problems which can make accurate diagnosis difficult. It is also among victims of partial seizures that one is most likely to observe displays of bizarre, learned, culturally conditioned behavior.

Simple partial seizures. These seizures have been variously called focal, focal motor, or focal sensory seizures. Although the symptoms may be motor, autonomic, psychic, sensory, or a combination, they are all linked to the affected area of the brain. The patient does not lose consciousness as a general rule, and the attacks last no more than thirty seconds. One type of simple partial seizure has been called the "Jacksonian." It characteristically begins with the twitching of one foot or hand, and the patient retains consciousness. Until very recently, seizures were classed as Jacksonian even if the activity subsequently spread to both sides of the body and involved loss of consciousness. Today, however, such seizures are classed as partial but secondarily generalized.

Complex partial seizures. These are characterized by complex symptoms and, unlike simple partial seizures, by impairment of consciousness. Often the patient appears to be conscious but later has no recollection of the episode. These seizures are usually associated with the temporal or frontal lobe and often begin with an "aura" which warns of the impending attack. Auras may include any of a large variety of sensations. Some of those most commonly reported are nausea, faintness, dizziness, numbness of the hands, lips, and tongue, choking sensations, and chest pain. Less often, patients have reported visions, palpitation, or disturbances of smell or hearing. Some patients have sensations that may begin hours or even days before the seizure. These symptoms are called the prodrome and most often involve irritability or feelings of uneasiness. When psychomotor symptoms appear during a seizure, they are generally semipurposeful and inappropriate actions such as clumsily attempting to disrobe. Patients often stagger about uttering guttural sounds. Such behavior is often confused with psychiatric disorder and is often alarming to those present.

Partial seizures secondarily generalized. This type occurs when seizures with a focal onset spread throughout the brain and produce generalized tonic-clonic seizures. Because the generalized phase is so dramatic, patients and their families often overlook the focal onset. The presence of an aura indicates the presence of the focal onset and the need to observe the initial phase more closely.

In recent years, some authorities have included as epileptic a range of symptoms typified by alterations of consciousness, abdominal pain, nightmares, and even psychotic behavior, if they are accompanied by abnormal electroencephalographic changes. The recognition of these "borderlands of epilepsy" has made the differential diagnosis between hysteria and epilepsy more difficult. Some epileptics, for example, have experienced psychotic episodes in association with abnormal brain waves during otherwise asymptomatic periods between seizures (Dongier 1959).

Hysteria and Pseudoseizures

Epileptics as well as nonepileptics may experience seizures that are not associated with abnormal brain wave activity and that have no known physiologic cause. These pseudoseizures are often called hysterical seizures or conversion reactions. As with epileptic seizures, pseudoseizures have characteristics that appear repeatedly. Epileptics with pseudoseizures tend to exhibit the same signs and symptoms in the same sequence with each episode. Nonepileptics' symptoms may vary in site and nature if there are many episodes. Pseudoseizures, despite the fact that they are responsive to the social environment and appear to vary among cultures, are often very difficult to distinguish from epileptic seizures. Between 8 and 20 percent of epileptics with intractable seizures are thought to experience pseudoseizures in addition to their epileptic seizures, and it has been estimated that even experienced neurologists can identify pseudoseizures only 75 percent of the time (Lechtenberg 1984:174). Opinion is divided concerning the causes of pseudoseizures. Generally they are thought to be among the manifestations of hysteria and thus a psychological problem. Recently, there has been renewed interest in the idea that they have some neurological basis, but there are those who insist that they represent nothing more than malingering.

Though the concept is Egyptian, the term "hysteria" derives from the Greek *hustera* meaning uterus (Veith 1965). The Kahun medical papyrus written around 1900 B.C.E. contains references to a number of strange maladies caused by the wandering of the uterus. Included among the case histories are a woman who cannot see, a woman who cannot open her jaw, and a woman who will not quit her bed. Other, probably organic, gynecological conditions are also included. Hippocrates had an almost identical explanation for hysteria and advised spinsters afflicted with the disease to marry. The symptoms that Hippocrates associated with hysteria were shortness of breath and seizures.

Both the ancient Egyptians and Greeks sought a physiological explanation for a variety of ill-defined symptoms of women. Galen, in the second century c.e., recognized a class of patients with seizures of psychic origin. The three symptoms which he called hysterical were seizures, shortness of breath, and contractures of the limbs. He rejected the notion of a mobile uterus leaping about inside the body, believing this to be anatomically impossible. Rather he felt that sexual abstention by men or women would cause these symptoms. He described one case in which manipulation of an hysterical woman's vulva caused orgasm and a complete cure of her symptoms.

From the end of the Roman Empire until well into the Age of the Enlightenment, persons with unexplained seizures, paralyses, or anesthesias were suspected of having had communication with the Devil. By the early nineteenth century, hysterical symptoms were thought to be the outcome of an emotional or neurological disorder which predominated in idle, often dissatisfied, young women but were also found among men. Hysteria was said to manifest itself in vague aches and neurological disfunctions but most particularly in convulsions and spells of peculiar behavior. By the middle of the century, gynecological explanations became popular once again, and there developed among the new "scientific doctors" a definitely punitive attitude toward the "flighty" female patients who so obstinately refused to be cured. The famous gynecologist Alfred Hegar and his pupils performed ovariectomies in cases of intractable hysteria. A neurologist, Nikolaus Friedrich, would cauterize the clitorises of those patients whose sexual needs and desires he deemed immoderate. In 1866 Jules Falret, psychiatrist at Salpêtrière in Paris, wrote: "These patients are veritable actresses, they do not know of a greater pleasure than to deceive. . . . In one word, the life of the hysteric is nothing but one perpetual falsehood" (Veith 1965:211).

In 1882, one of the buildings at Salpêtrière was in such a state of disrepair that it had to be torn down and rebuilt. This provided an excuse for rearranging the inmates of the wards, and epileptics and hysterics were housed together. Hysterics from the lower classes were institutionalized for custodial care at that time, a situation which appears to have aggravated their symptoms. Jean Martin Charcot was given custody of the new ward and was soon impressed by the fact that the hysterics had "caught" epilepsy from their neighbors. Young women who had been paralyzed or blind were soon throwing fits all over the ward. Charcot called this condition "hystero-epilepsy" but then recognized that the hysterics were mimicking the epileptics. He, however, considered hysteria a neurological disease which manifested itself by mimicry, susceptibility to hypnosis, and a clear-cut, four-stage progression of severity ending in a full-blown convulsive picture. Charcot introduced some very fundamental ideas about hysteria which have been retained by all schools of thought. First, hysteria, like hypnosis, has some kind of neurological reality and represents a special state of consciousness. When a hysteric or hypnotized subject does not respond to a painful stimulus, he is doing more than acting as if he does not feel it; in fact, he does not feel it. Second, the hysteric, like the hypnotized subject, is very susceptible to external influences.

The respectability given to hysteria by Charcot stimulated research into the therapeutic use of hypnosis in hysteria. The idea was that, as almost everyone is more or less susceptible to hypnosis, hysteria is not a disease but a dysfunctional use of naturally high levels of suggestibility. This approach was further developed by Ernst Kretschmer, who believed that hysterics combined an innate tendency to retreat into instinctive, involuntary behavior with the will to be sick (Kretschmer 1926). At the present time, there is a renewed interest in the normal and pathological occurrence of the dissociative reaction, the psychological process that walls off certain activities from consciousness. Such common phenomena as absentmindedness, daydreaming, and "highway hypnosis" are examples of partial dissociative reactions (West 1967).

Hypnosis is another kind of dissociative state. Under hypnosis patients are able to undergo major surgery without anesthesia. Neurophysiologists have tried to elucidate the mechanism of hypnotic anesthesia without definitive results (Halliday and Mason 1963). One major problem is that there is no physiological sign associated with the presence of any dissociative state. There is, however, a subjective difference for the "counterfeit" and the "real" subject (Orne 1959). In withstanding pain, the "real" hypnotized subject is aware of the stimulus but is just not bothered by it. The "counterfeit" feels the pain but is determined not to show it. For this reason, it is very difficult to recognize whether a person is really hypnotized. And, for the same reason, it is not always possible to distinguish between a malingerer and a hysteric. Both, however, are clearly susceptible to their cultural milieu; the symptoms and the course of their "disease" ought to be subject to it.

Although Freud was well-trained in neurophysiology, he soon abandoned the search for the neurological roots of hysteria and concentrated on discovering causative factors in the psychosocial environment. He had briefly been a student of Charcot and had become interested in hysteria. When he returned to Vienna, he collaborated with Josef Breuer who had discovered that hysterics under hypnosis will recall some emotional past experience and be cured of their symptoms. Together they suggested a theory of conservation of psychic energy: An emotional drive which cannot express itself is converted into a physical symptom (Breuer and Freud 1937). In Freud's experience, patients who used hysterical symptom formation had invariably suffered some disturbance in the resolution of their Oedipal feelings.[2] All these patients' sexual drives had an incestuous taint for them and caused them anxiety. They dissociated the awareness of their sexual urge from their consciousness and attached their anxiety to a symptom with which they became preoccupied. The "primary gain" thus achieved is the reduction of anxiety achieved by converting the psychic distress into a more acceptable physical symptom which symbolically expresses the unconscious wish at the time it prevents it from being carried out. But as the symptom also brings a great deal of attention from relatives and friends, it also achieves a "secondary gain." These "conversion reactions," in Freud's experience, were found only among patients who experienced psychic trauma during the "phallic stage" during which time the Oedipal conflict is experienced. Patients whose development was abnormal during the earlier "oral" and "anal" stages preoccupied themselves, instead, with phobic ideas or compulsive behavior.

Though hysteria has been a recognized illness since ancient times, it has always been a poorly defined one. It has, however, always been thought of as a disease of younger women with seizures and spells of irrational behavior its important symptoms. In addition to the lack of agreement over the causes of hysteria there is also, at present, considerable confusion concerning the stability of the symptoms themselves. One common view holds that hysteria was more common in preindustrial societies and that seizures are no longer commonly seen among hysterical patients in the industrial societies of the West. The most recent edition of the *Diagnostic and Statistical Manual of Mental Disorders* (American Psychiatric Association 1980) avoids using the concept and the term "hysteria." Instead, the multiple meanings of the term have been included in new categories.

A long list of symptoms is included under the heading "conversion disorders" in the manual. The most obvious and "classic" of these are those that suggest neurological disease, such as paralysis, aphonia, seizures, coordination disturbances, akinesia, dyskinesia, blindness, tunnel vision, anesthesia, and paresthesia. More rarely, other systems are involved. Vomiting, as a conversion symptom, may represent revulsion and disgust, for example. And false pregnancy can represent both a wish for, and a fear of, pregnancy. The course of conversion disorder is not well known but is thought to be of short duration in most instances. In addition to prior physical disorders such as epilepsy, extreme psychosocial stress and exposure to others with real symptoms are thought to be predisposing factors. Also people with histrionic or dependent personalities are more susceptible than others.

Epidemiology

Epilepsy. The first question we address is whether the Navajos' concern about seizures is the result of their having suffered more from epilepsy than the Pueblos. Do the Navajos have some genetic characteristic that makes them more susceptible to seizures? Were the living conditions of the village-dwelling Pueblos so much better that their children were less likely to be damaged at birth or exposed to the infections that cause epilepsy, or were Navajo adults more at risk for head trauma as the result of hunting accidents and the like? Although we can never know the answers to these questions, depending as they do on knowledge of the unrecorded past, there are several reasons to doubt that either genetic or environmental differences were sufficient to have had an appreciable affect on the belief systems. Of overriding importance is the fact that members of small societies cannot have enough direct experience of low-frequency phenomena like epilepsy for them to react in a manner different from a group with even half the incidence. The Navajos, for instance, continue to believe that suicide is committed by the sick, the aged, and the socially isolated, although in reality the vast majority of suicides are committed by young married males (Levy 1965). Direct observations are explained as "unusual" and do not "falsify" belief.

Aboriginally, Pueblos practiced village endogamy which produced small, inbreeding populations. The Zunis and Hopis are still considered genetic isolates, and their rates of albinism are among the highest in the Western Hemisphere (Jones 1964; Woolf 1965). The Navajos are not thought of as genetically isolated, although some Navajo subpopulations show considerable inbreeding. They are also measurably different from the Pueblos despite some three hundred years of contact and intermarriage (Spuhler and Kluckhohn 1953). If heritability explains differences in epilepsy rates, these differences should be discernible today and Navajo rates should be higher than Peublo rates to account for the Navajos' concern about seizures. But epilepsy has also been called a poor man's disease because harsh living conditions expose individuals to a large variety of conditions that predispose to epilepsy. As American Indians are among the nation's most poverty-stricken minorities, epilepsy should be more prevalent among them than it is in the general population.

During the past twenty years, several good epidemiological surveys of epilepsy made in Iceland, England, and the United States report crude prevalence rates between 3.6 and 5.5 per 1,000 population (Kurland, Kurtzke, and Goldberg 1973). Epidemiological studies of epilepsy, however, are plagued by a variety of problems. Of prime importance in this regard is the lack of agreement on the definition of epilepsy itself, as well as on what constitutes an active or an inactive case. In addition, there are difficulties involved in estimating the size of the population universe, and the number of cases not identified by the case-finding procedure. The most rigorous survey conducted in a community in the United States was done in Rochester, Minnesota, by W. Allen Hauser and Leonard T. Kurland (1975). We adopted their criteria and definitions so that our findings would be comparable with theirs.

All patient contacts in the Indian Health Service, whether in an IHS or contract facility, are recorded in a computerized data retrieval system. All patients living on the Hopi or Zuni reservations, in any of the Tewa Pueblo villages, or in the Tuba City Service Unit on the Navajo reservation who received a diagnosis of any seizure or hysterical disorder between July 1, 1971, and June 30, 1978, were identified.[3] All psychophysiologic disorders were also identified. The medical charts of individuals so identified were reviewed to verify tribal affiliation, to see if they met the criteria for a diagnosis of epilepsy or hysteria, and to see whether they could be classed as "active" cases. Field interviews with the families of epileptics and with knowledgeable members of the community then sought to find epileptics not already identified. The interviews were extensive among the Tewas and Zunis, less so among the Hopis and Navajos. This procedure did not identify any new cases qualifying for inclusion in the study.

Following Hauser and Kurland, we accepted as epileptics all individuals who had historical or clinical evidence of at least two convulsions occurring at two different times which were not caused by an identifiable metabolic or acute structural ab-

normality. The presence of an epileptic seizure was accepted if
(a) the seizure was known by history and there was an abnormal electroencephalogram, (b) if the seizure was observed by a
physician who believed it to be epileptic, and (c) if the seizures
were known by history only but responded to antiepileptic
medication. Individuals were included as "suspected" epileptics if, after a single seizure, a physician judged them to be at
risk for further seizures and placed them on medication even if
there was no recurrence of seizures. Excluded from consideration were (a) single, untreated seizure episodes with no known
cause; (b) single and multiple seizure episodes associated with
an acute illness; (c) seizures associated only with febrile illness
regardless of elaborateness or frequency.

Prevalence day was December 31, 1976. Only individuals
who were alive on that day and had experienced seizures or had
been on medication during the five-year period January 1, 1972,
through December 31, 1976, were included.[4] There were a
number of epileptics in each tribe who had died prior to prevalence day. There were also seven Navajos and six Hopis who
were possibly epileptic but who were not included in the analysis. These patients' charts contained no description of the seizures, no indication of how or by whom the diagnosis was
made, and no evidence that antiepileptic medication either
controlled seizures or was taken during the study period. These
patients were, however, treated as epileptics by physicians
(Table 4.1).

The crude prevalence rate of epilepsy in Rochester was 5.7
per 1,000 population. The age-adjusted rates per 1,000 population for the four Indian tribes were significantly higher: Tewas,
7.5; Navajos, 8.2; Hopis, 8.0; Zunis, 9.1 (Table 4.2).[5] Environmental factors accounted for the difference between Indians
and non-Indians. The Indians had significantly more epilepsy
attributed to trauma, postencephalopathy, and inflammatory
disease (Tables 4.3 and 4.4). Almost all the cases due to trauma
resulted from accidents sustained while intoxicated, and almost all the cases of postencephalopathic epilepsy were consequent on many years of excessive drinking.

Epilepsy resulting from inflammatory disease was also significantly higher among the Indians. Navajos and Hopis, and

Table 4.1. Disposition of Cases

	Navajo	Hopi	Zuni	Tewa
Active epileptics: *In study*				
Seizures between 1/1/75 and 12/31/76	66	29	41	14
Seizure-free 2 yrs. and not on medi- cation	4	3	3	4
Seizure-free 2 yrs. on medications	9	7	4	
Seizure-free 5 yrs., on medica- tions, multiple seizures prior to control with medications	5	1	1	
Suspected epilep- sy (single seizure, on medication)		2	1	1
TOTAL	84	42	50	19
Possible epilepsy: *Not in study*				
Remission: sei- zure-free 5 yrs., not on medica- tions, seizures recur after preva- lence day			1	
As above, sei- zures do not recur after preva- lence day	4	3		2
Inadequate chart but treated as epileptic	3	3	6	2

Table 4.2. Prevalence Rates per 1000 Population in Rochester, Minnesota, January 1, 1965, and in Indian Tribes, December 31, 1976

Age	Rochester	Navajo	Hopi	Zuni	Tewa
0–9	3.3	4.4	5.0	5.0	8.3
10–19	4.4	12.3	7.6	6.5	8.0
20–39	6.0	10.4	6.7	7.6	7.4
40–59	7.3	8.2	7.2	13.6	8.4
60+	10.2	4.9	10.4	18.5	4.2
Crude rate	5.7	8.4	8.0*	7.9	7.6
Age adjusted rate		8.2		9.1	7.5
Cases	268	84	42	50	19
Total Population	46,650	10,000	6,200	6,300	2,500

SOURCE: Hauser and Kurland (1975:25).
*Rate adjusted from 6.9 to account for estimated number of cases in group of missing medical charts.

Table 4.3. Etiology of Epilepsy

Etiology	Rochester	Indian
Vascular	27	11
Traumatic	27	36
Inflammatory	15	25
Neoplastic	21	1
Postencephalopathic	20	19
Intrauterine	7	6
Degenerative	3	1
Unclassifiable	9	3
Cause undetermined*	387	93
TOTAL	516	195

SOURCE: Hauser and Kurland (1975:33, Appendix Table 2).
*Hauser and Kurland do not enumerate these cases. We have assumed they equal the total number of cases, less those classed by cause.

Table 4.4. Chi-square Analysis of Etiologies
Rochester versus Indians (df = 1 in all cases)

Etiology	Chi square	Probability
Vascular	0.03	>0.8
Traumatic	5.1	0.02
Inflammatory	6.0	0.01
Neoplastic	0.0*	1.0
Postencephalopathic	9.4	<0.01
Intrauterine	2.25	>0.1
Degenerative	2.0*	>0.1

*Chi square corrected for continuity.

North American Indians generally, are known to have high rates of bacterial meningitis, especially meningitis due to *Haemophilus influenza* (Coulehan et al. 1976; 1981).[6] The occurrence of neurological sequelae including seizures is also high, but whether this is because the disease occurs more frequently, earlier in infancy, or because there is a delay in diagnosis is not yet clear. In sum, the higher rates of epilepsy among Navajos as well as Pueblos are best explained by environmental factors associated with poverty, alcoholism among adults, and bacterial meningitis among infants. That the rates did not differ appreciably among the four tribes convinces us that the reason for the cultural importance accorded seizures by the Navajos is not a higher susceptibility to the disease.

Hysteria and pseudoseizures. Since there is no agreed-upon definition of hysteria, it is almost impossible to compare the results of one study with those of another or to take the results of any very seriously. German and Scandinavian surveys suggest that the prevalence of hysteria may be anywhere from 1.1 to 5 per 1,000 population over the age of ten (Ljunberg 1957), and a rate of 4 was reported for Nova Scotia (Leighton et al. 1963). These findings suggest that hysteria may be about as prevalent as epilepsy.

Current opinion is that the classically described symptoms

of conversion hysteria—convulsions, paralyses, anesthesias, et cetera—have given way to psychophysiological disorders over the past eighty years. Contemporary clinical evidence suggests that pain and simulated bodily disease are now the most frequently seen forms of conversion reaction (Nemiah 1967). Changing styles of diagnosis and increasing sophistication of hospital staffs may account for much of the perceived change, however. What was once diagnosed as hysteria may today be classed as a "psychophysiologic disorder," a category which came into use only with the emergence of "psychosomatic medicine" during the years preceding World War II.

That the classic form of conversion reaction is still with us, however, is evidenced by a number of studies that report rates of conversion hysterias seen in large urban hospitals which range from 2.7 per 1,000 outpatient visits to 8 per 1,000 hospital discharges per year (Lewis and Berman 1965; McKegny 1967). More recently, a survey in northern India identified an 8.9 per 1,000 prevalence of "ever having suffered" from hysterical seizures (Dube and Kumar 1974), while a comparative study of the incidence of new cases of conversion hysteria in Monroe County, New York, and Iceland showed an incidence of 22 and 11 per 100,000 per year, respectively (Stefansson, Messina, and Meyerowitz 1976).

Epidemics of hysterical conversion reactions have also been reported over the past forty years (Johnson 1945; Knight, Friedman, and Sullianti 1965; Schuler and Prenton 1943). An epidemic of pseudoseizures among twenty-one girls and one boy, and another of one-sided tremors of the leg among high school students are reminiscent of the patients in Charcot's hospital ward in nineteenth-century Paris.

There is, nevertheless, evidence that the symptoms of hysteria vary from culture to culture. Abse believes that the classic forms of hysteria are still common in the rural south (Abse 1959:287). The hysterical seizure is thought to be a less sophisticated form of somatization and, therefore, more likely to be found among the less well educated. In Appalachia, for example, from 25 to 30 percent of hospitalized patients are said to show manifestations of hysterical seizures at some time during their hospitalization (Weinstein, Eck, and Lyerly 1969). Of six-

teen men who displayed these symptoms, twelve had later-
alized motor and sensory involvement of a limb or one side of
the body. Hallucinatory experiences included seeing dead people, perceiving that someone was trying to kill the subject, and
thoughts of a nephew killed in Iwo Jima. During the Second
World War, pseudoseizures were found more frequently among
troops of the Indian Army than among British soldiers (Abse
1950). At the other extreme, a study of psychiatric disorders in
the Virgin Islands found no cases of conversion reaction among
the Islanders, although cases were found among patients from
Cuba and other countries (Weinstein 1962:185–86).

We reviewed the charts of all individuals receiving a diagnosis of any type of hysteria, hyperventilation of psychogenic
origin, or physiologic disorder of probable psychogenic origin.
Of these, only patients with symptoms consistent with a diagnosis of hysteria occurring during the five years prior to prevalence day were analyzed.

Within the general category of hysteria, diagnostic styles
seemed to vary among hospitals. Episodes, by description identical to those diagnosed as pseudoseizures in the Tuba City
hospital, were more often simply called "hysterical reactions"
in Keams Canyon and Santa Fe. To make the task of comparing
cases from all these hospitals easier, we sorted the cases to conform to the style used in the Tuba City hospital.

More diagnoses were made among the Navajos (28) than
among the Pueblos (23), yielding rates of 2.8 and 1.5 cases per
1,000 population, respectively. The difference is significant and
is accounted for by the fact that nine of the Navajo hysterics
were epileptics. When epileptics with pseudoseizures are left
out of the calculations, the levels of hysteria are almost the
same in both groups: Navajo, 1.9; Pueblo, 1.5 (per 1,000).

Epilepsy combined with hysteria accounted for 11 percent of
the 84 Navajo epileptics. There were four cases of pseudoseizures, one of hysterical paraplegia, and four cases listed only as
"suspected hysterical overlay," a term indicating, we believe,
that the physician was not able to observe the seizures suffi-
ciently to determine whether there were true pseudoseizures
in addition to the epilepsy. The percentage of hysteria among
Navajo epileptics is significantly higher than among the

Pueblo epileptics, among whom no pseudoseizures were recorded, although one Pueblo epileptic had a diagnosis of hysterical reaction which was not described.

In the general population, between 8 and 20 percent of patients with intractable seizures are said to have pseudoseizures in addition to their epilepsy (Lechtenberg 1984:177). Because antiepileptic medication can eliminate or decrease the frequency of most types of seizures, persistently poor seizure control despite good compliance may be called intractable. But to make such a determination, the physician must have sustained contact with and knowledge of the patient. The epileptics in this study cannot be classed by these criteria with any degree of confidence. Rather, it seemed to us that the psychological problems contributed to the patient's noncompliance so that a true measure of intractability was unattainable.

There was no difference in the proportions of all conversion reactions or of pseudoseizures among the two groups. Hysterical blindness or paralysis is as alarming as a seizure and as likely to be brought to the attention of a physician. Pseudoseizures and other forms of conversion hysteria accounted for 61 percent and 18 percent of the 28 Navajo cases of hysteria, respectively, while among the Pueblos the comparable figures were 61 and 13 percent.

The descriptions of pseudoseizures found in the medical charts led us, at first, to believe that Pueblos tended not to emulate major seizures and might exhibit more restrained motor activity than the Navajos. Pueblo patients were described as going rigid and remaining immobile, or fainting and becoming unresponsive. To determine whether the difference was real, seizures were classed as either "active" or "passive," depending upon the extent of motor activity involved. Only 29 percent (4) of the 14 Pueblo patients with pseudoseizures were classed as "active" compared with 59 percent (10) of the 17 Navajos with pseudoseizures. Although seeming to confirm our impressions the difference was not, however, statistically significant (chi square corrected for continuity = 1.75; df = 1; p = .2).

In several respects Navajo and Pueblo hysterias were much like those found in the general population. Very much an affliction of women, only 4 percent of Pueblo and 14 percent of

Navajo hysterics were male. For the majority of patients the symptoms were transient and, over time, each patient displayed a variety of symptoms. Young women whose attacks began in late adolescence would, most often, become free of their hysterical symptoms after marriage and the birth of children. Pueblo hysterics were very unlike their Navajo counterparts in respect of age at onset, however. The average age at onset for Navajos was 21.3 years compared with 29.7 years for the Pueblos. Navajos tended to have their first hysterical episode before age twenty and only 18 percent had their first experience after age thirty. By contrast, 48 percent of the Pueblo hysterics were thirty or older when they had their first hysterical attack. These women tended to have episodes of fainting or going rigid associated with the death of a loved one. Some Zunis were brought to hospital after attending a funeral for a husband or son. Hopi women would collapse on hearing of the death of a son. Cases of suicide especially seemed to precipitate acute hysterical reactions. This pattern may be related to the Pueblo belief that the spirit of the deceased child or spouse tries to "take" the subject with him to the other world. In earlier times, there were no public funerals. The body was quickly buried by a few male relatives, who subsequently underwent a purification ceremony. The comportment of survivors were always restrained and dignified at these times. It is possible that, as burial customs changed, a new pattern appropriate to mourning emerged. Nevertheless, our impression is that the cases brought to the attention of physicians are those with a variety of personal and family problems and represent true hysteria. In part, the difference in age of onset is accounted for by the seven Navajo epileptics whose pseudoseizures started very soon after their epilepsy. Nevertheless, there seems to be a real difference in the dynamics of hysteria among the two groups.

Psychological problems. To further test the idea that Navajo beliefs about incest and seizures rather than a general Navajo propensity to hysterical disorders are the cause of the pseudoseizures experienced by Navajo epileptics, we hypothesized that the family of a Navajo child with epilepsy would withdraw emotional support and thus create emotional disturbance soon after the onset of the disease. Further, we suspected that community disapproval would intensify these problems during adolescence and early adulthood, making adjustment to adult life very difficult.

From the total of 84 Navajos and 111 Pueblos identified as active epileptics, we selected all those patients whose epilepsy started before age twenty, whose convulsions were not the direct consequence of a preexisting emotional problem (i.e., excessive drinking leading to head trauma), and who were not also retarded. The latter exclusion was made because most moderately and severely retarded children are institutionalized and because their emotional problems might be more closely associated with their retardation than with their seizures. From the population of identified epileptics, a study group of 46 Navajos and 42 Pueblos was obtained.

As predicted, Navajos were found to have social and emotional problems more often (p = < .05) than did Pueblos (Table 4.5).

To compare the age of onset of psychological problems among the two groups and for all subsequent comparisons, all individuals aged 0–5 years were excluded from consideration. There were three Pueblo children under six years of age who were said by their mothers to cry easily or to be quick to anger. These minimal complaints may persist, but, as so few Navajo preschoolers had good contact with the medical system, our data on them were lacking and we felt that noting problems at

Table 4.5. Prevalence of Emotional and Social Problems Among Epileptics With Age of Onset Less Than 20 Years

Problems	Navajo	Pueblo	Total
Present	28	16	44
Absent	18	26	44
TOTAL	46	42	88

Chi square = 4.55; df = 1; p = < .05.

Table 4.6. Age at Onset of Problems, Individuals Over Five Years of Age

Age at Onset	Navajo	Pueblo	Total
0–13 years	11		11
14–19 years	17	13	30
TOTAL	28	13	41

Fisher's Exact Test: p = <.05

this age would bias the findings. Navajos were found to exhibit problems prior to age 14 significantly more often (p = < .05) than the Pueblos (Table 4.6).

Most of the individuals identified as having psychological problems had at least one, either over time or at a given time. All psychotic disorders were classed as severe, as were pseudo-seizures, hyperventilation, and hysterical reactions (if there was a history of many episodes over a period of a year or more for these three neurotic disorders): suicide attempts, murder, attempted murder, and death by murder (when other problems were also present); and chronic alcoholism. Classed as mild were single episodes of hyperventilation, a diagnosis of "hysterical overlay," withdrawn behavior, neurotic depression, manipulative behavior, suicidal ideation, aggression, drinking bouts, and any single episode of drug overdose in the company of friends (Table 4.7). Although males in the two groups did not differ, significantly more Navajo females had severe problems than did Pueblo females (p = < .05; Table 4.8).

Only Navajos (two males and one female) were diagnosed as psychotic. Only Navajos were involved in homicide or homicide attempts: two females were murdered, one male murdered by his brother, and another was seriously stabbed by his brother. Only Navajos (two males and one female) made serious suicide attempts. Seven Navajo women were diagnosed as having persistent hysterical reactions and another had a few isolated episodes. One Pueblo male also had a few episodes.

Table 4.7. Clinical Description of Individuals With Psychological and Emotional Problems
(arranged by tribe, sex, age at prevalence day, and severity of problem)

Navajo Males

6–13 years

Severe 1. Childhood psychosis, crying jags, hits head on wall, kids throw stones at him.

Mild 2. Shy, lonely, does poorly in school, in special education.
3. Anxious and depressed, in special education.
4. Depressed, lonely, misses father he has never seen.
5. Very hyperactive, bizarre behavior at age 13, confused states, stress at school.

14–19 years

Severe 6. Attacks mother, hits showers, starts heavy drinking at age 18.
7. Problems with family start at age 14, binge drinking, suicide attempt at age 18, murdered his brother at age 20.
8. Suicide attempt with gun at age 20.
9. Rebellious between ages 14 and 19, problems with family, possible hysterical overlay after age 20, stabbed by brother.
10. Lives with grandparents between ages 14 and 19, severe alcoholism after age 20.

Mild 11. Hyperactive, hostile, aggressive, starts fights at school, seizures and behavior problems at age 14.
12. Dislikes school and wants to stay home.

Pueblo Males

14–19 years

Mild 1. Excessive drinking.
2. Hostile and aggressive.
3. Anxiety reactions, possible hysterical seizures.

20+ years

Severe 4. Alcoholism.
5. Chronic alcoholism.
6. Severe alcoholism.

Table 4.7. (*Continued*)

Navajo Females

6–13 years

Severe 1. Manipulative, fears loss of love, nightmares, somatic complaints, hysterical seizures at age 13, sent on LDS (Mormon Church) placement at age 14.
2. Severe emotional problems, maintained on Thorazine.

14–19 years

Severe 3. Severe psychological problems, hysterical episodes between age 6 and 13, hyperventilation after age 14.
4. Isolated by overprotective family until age 13, then aggressive at home and school, siblings leave home to avoid her, becomes promiscuous, has illegitimate child, raped and murdered at age 19.
5. Between 14 and 19 years of age possible hysterical overlay, killed, murder suspected.

Mild 6. Isolated, lonely girl kept out of school by mother.
7. Before age 13, withdrawn and depressed, after age 14 problems with family.
8. Easily angered, does poorly in school, in special education, seeing psychologist.

20+ years

Severe 9. Between age 14 and 19 suicide attempt, complex hysterical disorder, hysterical overlay after age 20.
10. Hysterical seizures between ages 14 and 19, acute alcoholism after age 20.
11. Between age 14 and 19 taken out of 6th grade by mother, promiscuous, has illegitimate child, multiple social problems after age 20, unspecified psychiatric disorder.
12. Pseudoseizures before age 19, then hysteria, multiple pseudoseizures and somatic complaints, on Thorazine.
13. Unhappy and maladjusted before age 20, then hysterical neurosis, psychotic depression, anxiety states, somatization, and hallucinations.

Table 4.7. (*Continued*)

Pueblo Females

14–19 years

Mild   1. Drug overdose in company of friends, does not take medications.

       2. Manipulative behavior, poor compliance, illegitimate pregnancy.

20+ years

Severe 3. Albino, exogenous depression, 20-year history of pseudoseizures, hyperventilation, hysterical reactions and anxiety states.

Mild   4. Anxiety reactions, hyperventilates after arguments.

       5. Suicidal ideation, neurotic depression, problems at home.

       6. Drinks, fights with father, arrested for driving while intoxicated.

Table 4.8. Severity of Problems, Individuals Over 5 Years of Age

Problems	Navajo	Pueblo	Total
MALES *			
Severe	6	3	9
Mild	9	4	13
Total	15	7	22
FEMALES +			
Severe	10	1	11
Mild	3	5	8
Total	13	6	19

---

*Chi square corrrected for continuity = .351; df = 1; p = < .5.

+Chi square corrected for continuity = 3.893; df = 1; p = < .05.

Attitudes. Interviews with parents revealed different ways of reacting to and dealing with the epileptic child. There were overprotective parents in both groups, though the overprotective Navajo parent tried to keep the child in isolation, an impossibility for the village-dwelling Pueblos. The characteristic reaction of Navajo parents to the epileptic child was withdrawal. One boy told us his parents would leave home for hours whenever he had a convulsion. In consequence, preschool-age Navajo children tended to be brought to hospital for treatment of seizures less frequently than Pueblo children. Children of school age were most often monitored and given medication by school nurses and counselors who maintained contact with the hospital.

By contrast, Pueblo parents tried to treat the epileptic child as normally as possible. They took special pains to talk with their own and their neighbors' children, so that they would react calmly when witnessing a convulsion and would not tease. Pueblo children, in consequence, developed normally until they were old enough to realize that their seizures made them different from other children. This usually occurred in junior high school, and it is at this time that numerous problems came to the surface. The outward placidity of Pueblo parents masked a tendency to deny the serious and chronic nature of the disease. The child was brought to hospital when seizures occurred, but the parents were resistant to the idea that the epilepsy might be a chronic condition which the child would ultimately have to cope with on his own. By treating the child as normal, Pueblo parents avoided dealing with the medical and social problems posed by the disease. By not speaking about the disorder with their epileptic child and not answering his questions, Pueblo parents provided the child with few means of coping as he became more independent in the adolescent period. After the age of fourteen, Pueblo epileptics began to experience emotional problems with the same frequency, if not the same degree of severity, as did the Navajos. Neither group was well maintained on medications, and seizures tended to recur frequently as a result. In effect, Pueblos were not "better" patients than Navajos, despite the more placid atmosphere that surrounded them.

Summary

The idea that Navajos have a predisposition to dissociative reactions because of their belief in possession and their individualistic, "Dionysian" temperament was not confirmed by the epidemiological data. Hysteria was more prevalent among the Navajos only because a high proportion of Navajo epileptics suffered pseudoseizures. Navajo epileptics also had more psychological and social problems. We interpret this to mean that the difference between the two groups in this regard is due to the Navajos' negative beliefs and attitudes toward seizures and not to a different personality configuration.

CHAPTER 5

Navajo Diagnosis

and Treatment

Navajos, we have seen, class their diseases by cause rather than by symptoms and, in theory, Navajo diagnosticians have no prior knowledge of the patient's symptoms or of the events surrounding the onset of his illness. We have also had occasion to note that asymptomatic individuals may think they are suffering from a seizure disorder if they believe they have been exposed to the causal agent, and individuals with a variety of organic conditions were often thought to have a seizure disorder. If patients are diagnosed according to the dictates of theory, there ought to be no measurable association of specific symptoms with any particular supernatural cause.

The association of etiological factors with symptoms, though loose, nonetheless exists (Wyman and Kluckhohn 1938). Some etiological factors may cause almost any symptoms, others a limited number. Most often a supernatural cause is thought to produce a variety of symptoms with one or two salient. Conversely, the same symptoms may result from one of several etiological agents. The question arises whether there is a nosology of diseases based on symptoms and syndromes and, if there is, how it may be discovered. We have noted that Navajo tradition clearly links three well-described seizures with three specific causes and ceremonial cures. In order for the connection to be made, however, the method of diagnosis must be less "magical" than represented. In fact, we find that patients and their families often dispense with diagnosticians altogether, believing that their knowledge of the events precipitating the condition is an adequate indicator of the cause. We also suspect that, in chronic cases, the hand tremblers have prior knowledge of the case, so that they diagnose and prescribe the appropriate

ceremonial cure. At the same time, however, the reluctance to
diagnose shameful etiologies like moth madness creates a situation in which seizure patients are treated by a variety of less
dangerous sings before one specifically for the cure of seizures is
tried.

Seizures and Other Disorders

To determine whether the forty epileptics and hysterics
studied in 1964 were diagnosed and treated differently from
others, we have compared them with two groups of patients.
The first, a "control" group of average Navajo patients, was
studied by Levy and Parker in 1962.[1] The distribution by age
and sex of this group approximated that of the total Navajo
population, as did the disease profile. Medical charts and healing ceremonies were recorded for the five-year period 1956–
1960. Few children had ceremonies performed for them, and
many adults had either not been sick at all or had had only one
or two ceremonies during the five-year period. The second
group consisted of thirteen elderly people who were clinically
depressed. A 50 percent random sample of residents of the
Tuba City Service Unit who were sixty-five years or older in
1982 was studied by Levy and Kunitz (1986). Of a total of 271
individuals, 23 were clinically depressed and, of these, 13 had
sings performed for them during the five-year period prior to
interview. The salient symptom of depression is dysphoria and
although mental confusion and forgetfulness may also be present, the condition is primarily a disturbance of affect rather
than of the cognitive process as is the case with seizures. By
comparing cases of depression with those of seizures, we hoped
to see whether major affective disorders were distinguished
from seizure disorders and whether dysphoria was associated
with a specific ceremonial cure. Subsequent to these comparisons we wished to see whether discriminations were made
among epileptics and hysterics and among the three types of
seizures said to signal the presence of hand trembling, frenzy
witchcraft, and moth madness.

The seizures experienced by the forty individuals with epilepsy and/or hysteria were classed as generalized, complex partial, or simple partial whether epileptic or hysterical.

During the 1950s and 1960s, patients seen in the Indian Health Service hospitals where we did our work had to be referred to hospitals at some distance from the reservation for neurological evaluation. Physicians often felt justified in making a diagnosis solely on observation of the seizures and a physical exam. Patients often refused to be transported to another hospital and, in the event repeated electroencephalographic tracings were thought necessary, they frequently resisted staying in hospital long enough for them to be done. In consequence, our diagnostic criteria differed slightly from those used in the epidemiological survey.

A diagnosis of positive epilepsy was accepted if (a) the patient had at least one seizure observed by a physician who had pronounced it epileptic, and/or (b) the patient had clearly abnormal electroencephalogram (EEG), ictal or interictal, which was consistent in location with the clinical characteristics of his seizures.

Seizures were classed as probably epileptic when, in the absence of an EEG and an observed seizure, the patient had (a) a history of early onset of seizures and (b) consistent, long-term response to antiepileptic medication, and (c) a history of stereotyped generalized or partial seizures, and/or (d) neurological deficits that were consistent with localizing signs during the seizure.

A diagnosis of positive pseudoseizures was accepted if a patient had (a) at least one seizure observed by a physician who had pronounced it hysterical, and (b) an absence of epileptic criteria, and (c) no abnormal EEG.

Seizures were considered probable pseudoseizures when, in the absence of an observed seizure, the patient had (a) elaborate, nonstereotypic spells and (b) spells that had their onset during adolescence or adulthood.

Only fourteen of the twenty-nine epileptics met the criteria for a positive diagnosis. Eight of the eleven hysterics, on the other hand, presented no diagnostic problems.

Mothway is extinct on the reservation, and we were able to find only one ceremonialist who knew it and one woman who

had the ceremony performed over her around the turn of the
century. This posed a problem, because it complicated the task
of determining whether people with seizures were ever diagnosed as suffering from moth sickness and treated with the
appropriate ceremony. After some inquiry, however, we learned
that a short form of Mountainway which included the bé'ékǫ́ǫ́z
ritual was used as a substitute for Mothway.[2] The active etiological agent in Mountainway is Changing Bear Maiden, a being
who married Coyote and learned all his evil powers. The Whirling Coyote ritual and Rabid Coyote songs are also used as a
substitutes for Mothway, the reasoning being that Coyote is the
originator of all incest and sexual mania and that the use of
Coyote to symbolize all forms of sexual excess and witchcraft is
thus consistent. Coyoteway itself may also be used, but it was
almost extinct in the western part of the reservation. When
patients said they had a Coyoteway performed, they meant the
ritual or the songs mentioned above.[3]

The bé'ékǫ́ǫ́z ritual of the Mountainway is associated with
sexual excess generally but is said to be used primarily for diseases of the genitalia. Several epileptic women had it prescribed for them and the case of one is particularly interesting.
A thirty-year-old woman with epileptic and hysterical seizures,
as well as what may have been psychotic paranoid or complex
fugue states, was diagnosed by her grandfather, a retired hand
trembler and stargazer. No ceremonies had been performed, ostensibly because there was no husband to help financially, although it seemed to us the family was reluctant to have their
problems known in the community. According to the parents,
the woman had committed incest with a clan brother and had
sexual relations with a man who had not been purified after
hunting. The grandfather felt certain that she needed the
bé'ékǫ́ǫ́z ritual for her incest and the Mountainway in its full
nine-night form for her contact with the unpurified hunter.
The seizure symptoms, especially the incontinence, were said
to be the same as those suffered by Coyote after he committed
incest and after his seduction of Changing Bear Maiden.[4] The
myth of the bé'ékǫ́ǫ́z ritual told to us by the grandfather consisted of the seduction of the Changing Bear Maiden by Coyote,
although he insisted that she was Coyote's sister and not his

wife as is generally thought. He did this, we believe, either because of the tendency to telescope important elements in the
Coyote myths to demonstrate their applicability to the subject
at hand or because of the need to create satisfactory substitutes
for the extinct Mothway and Coyoteway.

Although said to be extinct in many areas of the reservation,
we were able to locate ten ceremonialists who performed
Frenzy-witchcraftway and several who performed Hand-tremblingway in the Tuba City area. The Turning Basket ritual was
used by one patient as a substitute for the Hand-tremblingway
while she was in hospital, although she had had Hand-tremblingway performed several times in the past, and by two patients to "restore their minds." Another patient used this ritual
specifically for a diagnosis of frenzy witchcraft. Although we
have seen the ritual performed, we are unable to place it in the
ceremonial system. The afflicted parts of the patient's body are
patted with the basket after a series of songs. The procedure is
not similar to the basket drumming used in many other ceremonials and the reference to turning or twirling seems to be a
direct reference to mental states.

We consider all of these ceremonies and rituals as specific
cures for seizure disorders. There are, however, other ceremonies which may be used by patients with seizures that do
not indicate the presence of an etiological factor primarily
thought to cause seizures. Themes of incest, sexual mania, improper unions, and evil females like Changing Bear Maiden and
Snapping Vagina are found in the myths of many ceremonials
and may be used by seizure patients as well as others. These
sings are analogous to a broad spectrum antibiotic. If one of
them cures the seizures, the need to diagnose an incest-related
etiology is avoided. These "nonspecific" ceremonies are Evilway, Enemyway, Black-Antway-Evil, the Windways, the Shoot-
ingways, Bigstarway, and Enemy Monster Way.[5] Flintway and
the Lifeways, because they are used for any chronic disorder,
have also been placed in this category.

There are also several sings which have none of these themes
in their myths of origin and which ought not to be used for the
treatment of seizures. The ceremonies used in the western
Navajo reservation which are in this category are Nightway,

Plumeway, Beadway, and Beautyway. The Blessingways, because they are not aimed at removing specific etiologic factors,
have not been included in the comparisons.

A sing was tabulated regardless of whether the diagnosis had
been made by a hand trembler or by the family. A sing was also
counted for the seizure patients if a diagnosis had been made
and the family was planning on having the ceremonial at the

Table 5.1. Ceremonies Performed for 20 Patients With Seizures, 208 Controls,
and 13 Depressed Patients
All ceremonies for the 20 patients with seizures were performed prior to
interview, 1964.
All ceremonies for the 208 controls were performed during the 5-year period,
1956–1960.
All ceremonies for the 13 depressed patients were performed during the 5-
year period prior to interview in 1982 or 1983.

Ceremonies	Seizure Patients		Controls		Depressed Patients		Total
	No.	%	No.	%	No.	%	
Specific for seizures	29	31			1	5	30
Nonspecific	61	64	132	94	17	85	210
Not for seizures	5	5	9	6	2	10	16
TOTAL	95	100	141	100	20	100	256

	Seizure Patients	Controls and Depressed Patients	Total
	No.	No.	
Specific for seizures	29	1	30
Nonspecific & not for seizures	66	160	226
TOTAL	95	161	256

Chi square corrected for continuity = 48.8; df = 1; p = < .0001.

Table 5.2. The Use of the Evilway Sings

Type Sings	Depressed Patients		Seizure Patients		Controls		Total
	Obs.*	Exp.†	Obs.*	Exp.†	Obs.*	Exp.†	
The Evilways	12	(6.9)	29	(32.7)	47	(48.5)	88
All Others	8	(13.1)	66	(62.3)	94	(92.5)	168
TOTAL	20		95		141		256

Chi Square = 6.46; df = 2; p = <.05.
*Obs. = Observed.
†Exp. = Expected.

time of interview. Sings were not counted if they were repeated for the second, third, or fourth time according to Navajo custom. Sings were recorded for twenty of the forty cases of epilepsy and hysteria. No ceremonies had been performed for ten individuals and no information was gathered for ten who were either children who had only epileptic seizures or alcoholics who developed seizures as adults.

Of all ceremonies performed for the epileptics and hysterics, 31 percent were those specifically for the cure of seizures (Table 5.1). By contrast, none of the control group and only one depressed patient were treated by ceremonies of this type. The difference between the seizure patients and the others is significant, and the probability of its happening by chance is less than one in ten thousand.

The depressed patients used the Evilways significantly more often than did others in the sample of elderly Navajos studied by Levy and Kunitz. This was also the case when the depressed group was compared with the controls and the seizure patients (Table 5.2). Epileptics and hysterics used the Evilways about as often as did the controls. The Evilways accounted for 60 percent of treatments among the depressed, almost twice the proportion of seizure-specific sings among the epileptics and hysterics. It would seem that other mental conditions are also

associated with specific ceremonial treatments, although there
is nothing in the myths or informants' accounts to suggest that
depression is anywhere defined as a disease.

Evilway is used to cure conditions caused by witchery and
ghost contamination. Both are said to cause loss of sleep, appe-
tite, and weight. Ghost contamination also produces a feeling of suffocation and "ugly" (hóchǫ́ǫ́) dreams, and witchery is
said to cause a "drying up." The myth of Evilway relates how
Coyote witched the hero by entering the bottom of his stom-
ach so that "his former thinking power was much weakened,
everything seemed to be beyond him . . . he could not even get
sleep. . . . Whatever he ate he always vomited. And too he began to wither away until he was aught else than skin and bone"
(Haile 1950:154–55). These are the salient somatic symptoms
of depression. The affective symptoms—dysphoria, feelings of
hopelessness, worthlessness, shame, and guilt—are made conspicuous by their absence.

A similar observation may be made about the symptoms of
mental disorder mentioned in the myth of Mountainway. This
chant is firmly associated with arthritis and mental disturbances, and there are many references to sore, aching, and
swollen limbs. We found only two passages which seemed to
refer to the cure of mental conditions, however. The first, recorded in the nineteenth century, says only, "But to him the
odors of the lodge were now intolerable and he soon left the
lodge and sat outside," and "The ceremony cured (him) of all
his strange notions and feelings. The lodge of his people no
longer smelled unpleasant to him" (Matthews 1887:410, 417).
In another recording of the myth we find, "Now the boy was
cured of all evil, and his old evil dreams; he had new thoughts
in a new body" (Wheelwright 1951:16). Despite the paucity of
references to mental states, however, Mountainway is a preferred treatment for anxiety, nervousness, fainting, temporary
loss of mind, delirium, violent irrationality, or insanity (Wyman 1975:19–21). It seems clear that depressed individuals as
well as those with seizures are sorted into groups according to
their symptoms. What is not apparent is why the symptoms of
mental disorder are not described in the myths of the sings
used to treat them and why, if depression is a circumscribed
syndrome, the Navajos do not identify it as a disease by name.

We believe, first, that Navajos avoid talking about mental conditions whenever possible, preferring to indicate the presence of an underlying mental disturbance by referring to physical symptoms which may or may not be caused by a mental malfunction. Secondly, we also believe that depression and hopelessness have a cultural importance for the Navajos equal to that of the major seizure, which makes it dangerous to objectify them in open discourse. The mind is thought to control the body: "All parts of man's body and spirit are coordinated by mind, will power, volition, reason, awareness" (Reichard 1963:34). Weakness of the body implies a mental disturbance. Thought and speech are also thought to have the power to create physical reality. The Navajo world was brought into being by supernaturals whose thoughts were realized through speech.[6] But, just as good thoughts and prayer compel the beneficent supernaturals, so also may evil be potentiated by bad thoughts and speech. Direct reference to the mental disturbance, then, makes it real. That Navajos find it preferable to refer to somatic symptoms suggests that the interaction between mind and body is not reciprocal but that the mind takes precedence.

A study of decisions to seek medical or ceremonial treatment made by members of the rural families in the control group over a two-year period revealed that complications of childbirth, broken and fractured bones, and lacerations were rarely treated by ceremonialists and never by them alone (Table 5.3). Conversely, the only symptoms treated exclusively by ceremonialists were faints and those instances in which the individual was asymptomatic but knew that he had contracted a Navajo disease (Levy 1983:143–44).

Psychiatrists and psychologists working with the Navajos have often commented on their tendency to somatize. Whether this is a correct observation or the consequence of a cultural style of communicating about mental distress is, we believe, a topic that deserves further study. In light of the discussion thus far it seems equally likely that Navajos are conditioned to present somatic symptoms and not thought or mood disturbances.

The fact that clinically depressed individuals were distinguished from others indicates that a distinction is made between emotion and intellect. Whether this discrimination

Table 5.3. Use of Physicians and Ceremonial Practitioners
for Self-Defined Illness Among 106 Individuals Over a
Two-Year Period

Symptoms and Conditions	Practitioner Consulted		
	Physician Only	Both	Ceremonialist Only
Childbirth and trauma*	23	7	0
All Others†	9	19	9

Chi Square = 19.6; df = 2; p = .001.
SOURCE: Levy (1983:144).
* Childbirth; prenatal and postnatal complications and examinations; fractures, lacerations, contusions.
† Problems of respiratory systems, including tuberculosis, pneumonia and upper respiratory infections; muscle and joint pain, including arthritis; deafness; crippling, including congenital hip displacement; blindness (cataracts); rashes, sores, and abscesses, including impetigo; diarrhea; faints; conditions ultimately diagnosed as diabetes, prostate infection, thrombosis, urinary tract infection, measles, and chicken pox; vague complaints and malaise; "lightning contamination" (no symptoms) and nightmares.

extends to other emotional disturbances cannot be inferred from the limited data at hand. What is clear, however, is that depressed individuals were quite willing to discuss their somatic complaints but, when pressed to talk about their mood, spoke only about their mental state in the most general way. They were extremely uncomfortable speaking about dysphoria. Rather than use the words for sadness ('ááh) and hopelessness (−chįį), they preferred to use the more general word yiniił (yini = mind or intellect + ił = in company with) which can mean worried, sad, or distraught depending on the context.

Depression, hopelessness, and loss of all pleasure and interest in life are a rejection of life, and Navajos are taught from childhood to resist such feelings at all cost. The central ceremony in the Evilway group is the Upward-reachingway (haneełnéehee), and it is tempting to think of this sing as "the upwardness of healing power" used to cure the "downward illness," depression, despite the fact that informants never referred to depression in this manner (Luckert 1981:ix). Depression is recognized nonetheless, and its victims are treated by the Evilways. Because the emotion is caused by "ugly" thoughts, volition is involved and depressed patients are ashamed of their feelings and try to hide them. It is as if the malady is equated with suicide in much the same way the Hopis consider those who lose the will to live to be suicidal. In the domain of mental illness, then, Coyote's qualities of chaos and excess produce the *tsi* behaviors, sibling incest, and seizures; his association with death and witchcraft produces "ugly" thoughts, or depression.

Discriminating Among Seizures

Turning now to the cohort of seizure patients, we find that discriminations are also made among epileptics and hysterics. Epileptics were treated with sings appropriate for their type of seizure significantly more often than were the hysterics (Table 5.4). But because so many individuals experienced more than one kind of seizure, it is of interest to focus attention on the seizures themselves. In this way, one can measure the extent to which all those with generalized seizures are treated with Coyote rituals regardless of their other seizures and ceremonial

Table 5.4. Patients Who Received Ceremonial Treatments Appropriate for Their Seizures (by diagnostic category)

Diagnostic Category	Treatments		Total
	Appropriate	Other	
Epilepsy	10	1	11
Hysteria	3	6	9
TOTAL	13	7	20

Fisher's Exact Test: p = .012.
NOTE: No information, 10; no treatments, 10.

Table 5.5. Treatment of Epileptics and Hysterics With
Seizure-Specific Sings (by seizure type)

	Yes	No	Total
Generalized seizures			
*and Coyote rituals**			
Epileptics	9	1	10
Hysterics	0	3	3
Total	9	4	13
Complex partial seizures			
and Frenzy-witchcraftway†			
Epileptics	4	1	5
Hysterics	2	3	5
Total	6	4	10
Simple partial seizures			
and Hand-tremblingway‡			
Epileptics	0	4	4
Hysterics	3	0	3
Total	3	4	7

*Fisher's Exact Test: p = .002.
†Fisher's Exact Test: p = .239.
‡Fisher's Exact Test: p = .028.

treatments. When analyzed in this manner, we can see that
epileptics with generalized seizures were treated with Coyote
rituals while hysterics were not (Table 5.5). Conversely, only
hysterics with unilateral seizures were treated with Hand-
tremblingway. Both complex partial seizures and hysterical
fugue states were treated with Frenzy-witchcraftway, however;
in the aggregate, there was no significant difference between
epileptics and hysterics, indicating that factors other than an
ability to distinguish the true epileptic from the hysteric are
involved.

We have seen that the Navajo epileptics identified by the epidemiological survey had more psychological and social problems than their Pueblo counterparts. This is also the case when

Table 5.6. Social Problems of Female Epileptics and
Hysterics Age Seventeen and Above (1964)

	Social Problems		
	Absent	Present	Total
Epileptic females	1	9	10
Hysteric females	7	3	10
TOTAL	8	12	20

Fisher's Exact Test: p = .01.

the epileptics in the group studied in 1964 are compared with
the hysterics. As there was only one male hysteric, the difference between groups is accounted for by the women. Significantly more epileptic than hysteric females had social problems (Table 5.6). Promiscuity and/or problem drinking were
noted for four epileptics and three hysterics. In addition, three
epileptics were prone to violent outbursts which may have
been caused by their disorder. What distinguishes them is the
number of epileptics who were raped, bore illegitimate children, or committed incest. When these problems are singled
out for consideration, the difference between the epileptics and
the hysterics is significant (Table 5.7).

Table 5.7. Incest, Rape, and/or Illegitimate Children Among
Female Epileptics Age Seventeen and Above (1964)

	Incest, Rape, and/or Illegitimate Children		
	Absent	Present	Total
Epileptic females	6	4	10
Hysteric females	10	0	10
TOTAL	16	4	20

Fisher's Exact Test: p = .04.

Of the 13 male epileptics, one had no problems and 2 were under seventeen years of age. The remaining 10 all had severe drinking problems. For 6, drinking was the only problem. The remaining 4 were also violent, and one had committed sibling incest. Whether this record indicates that male epileptics have more severe problems than nonepileptic males, however, is a moot question given that 75 percent of a sample of rural Navajo males living in the western part of the reservation exhibited drinking behaviors that the general population associates with alcoholism (Levy and Kunitz 1974).

The careers of epileptics continued to differ from those of the hysterics between 1965 and 1975. Only the 11 epileptics and 10 hysterics who lived in the Tuba City area were followed during this period. By 1975, 4 of the epileptics had died from unnatural causes. The only male to die had been suicidal since age sixteen, but whether his death was due to suicide or trauma incurred during a seizure was never determined. Two epileptic women were found dead after drinking, one from exposure, the other from undetermined causes. Both had histories of drinking and promiscuous behavior and had been diagnosed as psychotic. Both were from poor families who did not take care of them, and both had committed incest. A third woman was found dead at some distance from her home where she had been herding sheep. The cause of death was never determined. All but 2 of the remaining 7 epileptics continued to lead difficult lives characterized by recurring seizures, drinking, divorce, and in one case, promiscuity.

In 1975 only two epileptics seemed to be leading normal lives. One, a young woman, was put on antiepileptic medication by the time she was six years old after a history of febrile seizures between ages three and four. Although her parents were not really acculturated, her mother was a hospital employee and seizures had been well controlled on medication. With the exception of a brief period characterized by adolescent rebellion, when she took her medications erratically, this patient had no psychiatric or social problems.

The other well-adjusted epileptic was a male who had experienced seizures since age three. While in school, nurses administered his medications and his seizures were well controlled. His parents did not supervise him well at home, however.

When fourteen years old he sustained a concussion during a seizure. After that, his parents were careful to see that he took medications regularly. When we saw him again in 1975, he had been seizure-free for twelve years. He and his parents had a very warm and loving relationship. Nevertheless, at twenty-six years of age, he was still single, socially isolated, and, perhaps, slightly retarded.

While conducting the epidemiological survey of the Tuba City Service Unit in the summer of 1980, we entertained some doubts about the significance of the number of epileptics who had died and wondered whether the sample was large enough to warrant our belief that Navajo epileptics led difficult lives and tended to die young. These doubts, however, were quickly dispelled when two of the younger epileptics identified by the survey died—one under mysterious circumstances, the other a victim of homicide. Both deaths occurred after prevalence day and so did not appear in our tabulations.

Only one of the ten hysterics in the Tuba City area died, and death was from natural causes associated with old age. Four had been symptom-free for many years and were leading normal lives in 1975. One woman continued to experience hysterical seizures along with some new symptoms such as globus hystericus which she described as a lump in the throat and a choking sensation which kept her from speaking for varying lengths of time. The remaining four continued to have problems, but their pseudoseizures had disappeared and they reported, instead, persistent psychosomatic complaints.

In summation, the process of diagnosing and prescribing ceremonial treatments takes symptoms into account in a manner that sorts individuals with seizures into a general class of disorders characterized by extreme (tsi) behavior clearly separated from clinically depressed patients as well as a group of "typical" patients. Hysterics were also treated differently from epileptics, although it is not clear that this is due to an ability to distinguish seizures from pseudoseizures, the chronicity of epilepsy, or some other factors not elucidated by the method of analysis employed in this chapter. In order to investigate this question further, each of the three conditions—hand trembling, frenzy witchcraft, and moth madness—will be examined separately in succeeding chapters.

CHAPTER 6

Hand Trembling

Opinions about the nature of shamans are diverse but appear to fall into one of four categories: (1) the shaman is a psychotic or neurotic; (2) the shaman is a healed psychotic; (3) the shaman may be normal or abnormal; (4) the shaman is eminently normal. The idea that shamans are psychotics or neurotics has persisted from the nineteenth century to the present.[1] Alfred Kroeber, for example, believed that "Not only shamans . . . are involved in psychopathology, but often also the whole lay public of primitive societies" (Kroeber 1952:318). At the other extreme is Jane Murphy's conclusion that "the group of shamans that came to attention in the St. Lawrence study appeared to reflect the population as a whole in distribution of psychiatric symptoms. The well known shamans were, if anything, exceptionally healthy in this sense" (Murphy 1964:76). Among those who believe that shamans are normal are those who have observed that shamans tend to inherit the role from their families (Gubser 1965:156; Ksenofontov 1955:211–12; Spencer 1959:303).

Although there is a wealth of material describing shamanistic rituals and social roles the world over, there are few studies that examine the personalities of shamans both before and after their initiation into the healing role. Where such studies have been done, however, there seems to be some agreement that becoming a shaman solves some difficult personal problems. Okinawan and Korean shamans, for example, are said to be deviant personalities who led lives marked by failure in interpersonal relations prior to becoming shamans (Lebra 1969; Harvey 1979). A large study of 56 Japanese shamans, however, found that only 20 percent showed signs of personal pathology and that by far the largest proportion, 80 percent, acquired shaman status through apprenticeship (Sasaki 1969).

Closer to our area of interest is a study of thirteen Mescalero Apache shamans of whom none were found to have been identified as deviants by other Apaches or cured by another shaman prior to their own assumption of the role. On the other hand, the authors of this study seem to share Kroeber's view of primitive society when they assert that the Apaches as a group suffer from a hysterical personality (Boyer et al. 1964; Boyer 1979). The Navajo hand trembler may be called shaman because she performs her art while in a trance and is thought to be possessed while doing so. Like Korean and Siberian shamans, her initial trance experience is involuntary and thought to be an illness, unless the ritual which simultaneously cures and initiates is performed immediately. Unlike shamans elsewhere, however, the Navajo diagnostician does not make a journey into the spirit world nor is the presence of the intrusive spirit made known by strange speech or actions. Hand tremblers we have seen did not appear to dissociate. Their performances in fact appeared to us to be rather deliberate and the trembling controlled. We felt that the role of diagnostician could easily be filled by individuals with normal or histrionic personalities. It seemed possible that the hysterics whose episodes of conversion consisted of shaking or trembling in one arm might become hand tremblers and so obtain some relief from their seizures. We thought it unlikely, however, that either psychotics or epileptics would be able to perform adequately for any period of time. Whether they ultimately became hand tremblers or not, we thought that hysterics would be more likely to produce the positively valued unilateral trembling of the diagnostician than the generalized convulsion thought to be caused by incest.

Nine individuals experienced epileptic simple partial seizures or hysterical bouts of hand trembling. Two epileptics were dropped from consideration, one because the family were Peyotists and had not diagnosed their daughter, another because she spoke no Navajo, had been raised away from the reservation, and had no knowledge of Navajo belief. Two epileptics had simple partial seizures consisting of unilateral convulsions that started early in life. The family of one of these girls was poor and, although the father was a singer, no attempt to treat the seizures had been made. We have had occasion to mention this man as a person who thought that he was *diitła*.

He believed that his daughter's seizures as well as his own resulted from a mistake he had made while performing a sing. We
suspect the family wished to avoid drawing attention to their
problems and so refrained from having sings. Another young
woman had been paralyzed on the right side since infancy. She
was retarded and had committed incest. At no time did her
family believe that she had the gift of hand trembling.

One very acculturated young woman who had hours of trembling in both arms thought she should become a hand trembler.
Whether a more traditional family would have concurred we
have no way of knowing. In any event, her symptoms were extremely variable and she made no serious efforts to become a
hand trembler, although she spoke Navajo and had a traditional
grandfather with whom she was very close. We were, nevertheless, intrigued by the idea that bilateral trembling of the
extremities could be presented as hand trembling and later had
occasion to note that some participants in peyote meetings
would hold one arm to keep it from shaking. This was taken as
a sign that some malign influence was at work and that the
individual in question required special prayers. We discussed
these observations with a psychiatrist whose patients sometimes complained of uncontrollable shaking of one arm. Later,
on several similar occasions, he asked his patients to release
the afflicted arm and found that both arms began to shake. We
wondered whether cultural expectations could influence the
way seizures were perceived and presented.

The Epileptics

Carl was a youth whose major seizures, fuguelike behaviors,
and episodes of conventional hand trembling were difficult to
diagnose because of his alcoholism. When he was thirteen
years old, his father—a hard drinking, half Irish, half Navajo
heavy-equipment operator—was stricken with a cerebral hem-
orrhage in the boy's presence and died a few days later. After-
wards, Carl began crying about his father and dreaming that he
heard his father trying to speak to him. For the next few
months, he attached himself to his father's drinking compan-
ions, among whom was a singer whose protégé he became. He

soon developed the capacity to hand tremble. He went to sings and learned to do sand paintings. He was serious about this activity and told his brothers that he could foretell the future. He had a suitcase in which he kept some herbs and sand which he would sometimes spread out on the floor at home in order to make a sand painting. On one of these occasions the family noticed that while he was working his arm began to tremble. Rather than accepting this as a gift for hand trembling, the family felt he should see a physician. His interest in Navajo religion was poorly received by his nine acculturated brothers and sisters, although his mother covertly encourage him. "He was good at it," she told us. "All the time people asked for him to help with the sand paintings."

Carl withdrew from his peers who teased him about his interest in ceremonies. He showed no interest in girls and dropped out of school several times before leaving entirely. By age fifteen he had begun to drink heavily. He would also act strangely for hours even when sober. He would come home in an irritable mood, throw tantrums when his mother refused to lend him the truck, and hit his younger brother. He would wander about aimlessly and was, at times, unresponsive. Carl never became a hand trembler and his episodes of hand trembling seem not to have recurred after he began drinking.

At age seventeen, after drinking with his father's former friends, he came running home to where his mother was weaving. He fell down and began to shake and stiffen. He turned blue, and the family had great difficulty restraining him. A singer was called for, who administered herbal medicines after which he went into a deep sleep for hours. These generalized seizures continued for the next three years interspersed with episodes of bizarre behavior. Once his mother was watching him chop wood when suddenly he began to work at a very rapid rate. Although she told him he had chopped enough, he kept working faster and faster, refusing to stop. He then ran toward his mother with the ax, yelled suddenly and dropped the ax as he began to convulse.

Carl's relatives considered his fugue states and his seizures to be part of the same malady. He came, finally, to medical attention when an older brother tried to have him committed to an

insane asylum. He had been living with this brother when he
began to have auditory and visual hallucinations. He kept saying that his mother and little brother were coming after him and
that he could see them through the window. At times he would
appear to be talking with someone, but when asked with whom
he refused to answer. Once he left the trailer and walked about
restlessly all night. In the morning he was still seeing his mother and younger brother who, he was convinced, were lying on
the road with a car about to run over them. The brother, becoming frightened, called the police who took Carl to the hospital
where the diagnostic impression was "severe alcoholism with
alcoholic hallucinosis and alcoholic withdrawal . . . possible
schizophrenia in remission." After his return home he stopped
his drinking and for the year prior to our interview with him had
only experienced the epileptic generalized seizures.

The diagnostic difficulties this case presents need not detain
us. Of importance here is the fact that, although he experienced episodes of hand trembling, he never became a diagnostician. It seems likely that the drinking unmasked familial
epilepsy—a grandmother and cousin have seizures. In our
opinion the epilepsy coupled with the bizarre behavior would
have made it impossible for him to perform adequately as a
diagnostician even if the family had supported him in the en-
deavor which, we have seen, they did not.

His bouts of hand trembling stopped before he had his first
epileptic seizure some three years after his father's death. Not
until then was a diagnostician consulted who said that the
cause of the problem was contamination by the father's ghost.
A blackening ritual from Evilway was performed for this. Later,
another hand trembler diagnosed contact with the remains of
ancient Pueblos (anasázi), and a full Enemyway was performed.
Carl believed this diagnosis was correct because he had "found
a whole anasázi skeleton up in that cliff. We busted the skull
and took the rest of it to the trader. They connected all the rest
of the bones and put them into the case."

After his return from the hospital in 1963, a hand trembler
diagnosed witchcraft. A witch was said to be after both Carl and
his father whose death had already been effected. A Turning
Basket ritual with a Blessingway was performed. Soon after this,
a hated uncle died; the family were convinced that he had been

the witch. Carl's behavior was called *tsi'ndidáá jikéya*, referring to his running off into the countryside, and he was said to be suffering from frenzy witchcraft. This is a rather atypical case of this form of witchcraft, not only because males were the victims but because death was the desired outcome. Seemingly, the bizarre, dissociative behavior influenced the diagnosis, and the case will be reexamined in another chapter.

Mary, whose case shall receive more attention in the next chapter, was a young woman with generalized epileptic seizures and hysterical attacks that looked like complex partial seizures. Of interest in this context is the fact that, on one occasion after leaving hospital against medical advice, she began to hand tremble at home. Although she knew none of the prayers, she had observed hand tremblers called in to diagnose her condition and was able to give a convincing performance. She described a circle with her hand and said that this type of sing must be performed for her as soon as possible and that going to an off-reservation hospital for evaluation would cause her death within a month's time. Her father, a Chiricahua Windway singer, suspected that she was fooling but, not wishing to take chances, performed a Chiricahua Windway with a sand painting of the moon. During the ceremony, Parker saw her grab her father's clothing. She refused to loosen her grip and began thrashing about forcing her father to hold her down. Although her father was a singer, no one took the hand trembling to mean that Mary should become a diagnostician. At the time we felt that her problems were too incapacitating for her to succeed in such a demanding role.

The Hysterics

Turning now to the ten women and one man who had only hysterical pseudoseizures, we note that only two women experienced episodes of hand trembling. These women had both been professional hand tremblers and a third became a hand trembler some years after we conducted our survey in 1964. Their stories are of some interest, first, because all three rejected the role and, second, because we have knowledge of the lives of two of them before they were initiated.

Clarissa was an elderly Paiute Indian well over seventy years old in 1964. She was a member of the remnant of a southern Paiute band that once occupied much of what is now the Tuba City Service Unit. Officially classed as Navajos, this small group of families living near Tuba City are poor and are looked down upon by the Navajos. Though some still identify with the Paiutes in southern Utah and the older people still speak Paiute, they have adopted Navajo clans and kinship terminology. In their health behavior, dress, and everyday life they form a subculture of the western Navajo.

Clarissa became a hand trembler before she was thirty years old. She stopped practicing voluntarily, however, after violating a tabu during a Windway ceremony. She was advised by a singer who said she would be bothered by the disturbed hand trembler spirits if she persisted in practicing her calling. Despite this ritual precaution, however, she began to be bothered by attacks of uncontrolled hand trembling and, later, by episodes of bizarre behavior. The latter involved spells of irrationality, bizarre behavior, running off into the desert, and occasionally beating people with her cane. Because she was always helped by Twirling Basket and Hand-tremblingway prayers and songs, she never came to hospital for treatment.

In 1962 Clarissa entered the isolation ward with active tuberculosis. She became anxious and fearful that she would be sent away to a sanatorium, and during the night her arm began to shake uncontrollably. According to the attending physician, she was rational throughout but was unable to control the shaking of her arm. By coincidence, the ceremonialist who had treated her for these outbursts in the past was then a patient on the same ward and was prevailed upon to sing over her. Levy and Parker were present during the performance, which included some songs from Hand-tremblingway and patting her hand with a basket. Within minutes, the shaking stopped and Clarissa spent the rest of the night in peace. We suspected that she would not have experienced this episode if the singer had not been on the ward at the time. A year after our interviews in 1964, Clarissa died from natural causes.

Since Clarissa was nearly deaf, we were able to learn little from her about her early life. Nor were her adult grandchildren able to tell us much about how she became a hand trembler, how long she had practiced her art, or how successful she had been. Although she was cantankerous and irritable in old age, we do not know whether she had always been a difficult person.

Mildred was said to have been bothered by intermittent attacks of hand trembling throughout childhood. Her father and his two brothers were not only singers but also hand tremblers and stargazers. She married when she was sixteen years old and, a year later, gave birth to a stillborn child. By the time she was twenty-three she had given birth to three children and appeared happy except that her husband drank too much. At this time, her father began pressuring her to become a hand trembler. Finally, after three days of uncontrollable hand trembling, Hand-tremblingway was performed and she assumed her role as diagnostician.

A year later, in 1960, Mildred's husband of nine years left her for another woman; only a few months later, she gave birth to her fourth child. This baby was hydrocephalic and, despite hospital care, soon died. Mildred became convinced that the family of the other woman hated her and was trying to do her harm. Shortly after the baby's death in 1961, symptoms more severe than hand trembling began to appear. She had itching of the arms, abdominal pains, and some alarming bouts of altered behavior. She complained of feeling "funny all over," a weakness and trembling all over her body, and a fear that what she was experiencing might kill her. She saw soldiers in battle and marines fighting Navajos. She saw Navajo men (whom she knew) butchering sheep, who would then ride after her and try to kill her. Once she cried out like a *yei* (masked god). She had sings for these symptoms and, during one, she became convinced that one of the men present intended to kill her. She grabbed a gun and attempted to shoot him. She began to have spells of sitting motionless for long periods of time and was sent to an off-reservation hospital for evaluation.

After the death of the baby and the onset of her "spells," a second Hand-tremblingway was performed because her father thought she had violated her own power and that it was "turning back on her." As the spells worsened, she and her parents became convinced that the woman who had stolen her husband was working frenzy witchcraft against her and Frenzywitchcraftway was performed twice. When this didn't work, the diagnosis was switched to one of plain wizardry. The family of the other woman were simply out "to get them." A Hopi healer performed a sucking cure and extracted a wood louse from Mildred's body. This treatment, the family felt, helped for some time.

During her hospital stay, she was quite cooperative, without hallucinations, but nonoriented. She was still convinced that someone was after her, intent on doing her bodily harm. There were no seizures but she assumed catatonic positions on several occasions. She was discharged with a diagnosis of schizophrenic reaction, catatonic type.

When she returned home she found that her cousin had come home from a tuberculosis sanitorium and that she too had lost her husband. The cousin had been known as a drinker, and soon Mildred began to drink with her. Sometime in 1963, Mildred began to attend peyote meetings in an attempt to stop her drinking. Her parents, however, were very much against the peyote church and felt that it was worse than alcohol. Nevertheless, she managed to attend peyote meetings and to bring peyote home with her, where it was later discovered.

After a night at a peyote meeting, Mildred's parents found her at home in a catatonic state. It seems that this had happened before when she consumed peyote at home. According to Mildred, it was at this meeting that the Road Chief (leader) told her that her father had once denied she was his daughter. She recalled this incident from her childhood and remembered saying, "If I am not your daughter, I'll die, I'll die." The Road Chief wanted her to recall the event so that both she and her father could feel less anxious. She knew that her father was only joking but, at the same time, she took it seriously and felt her father was rejecting her. Again she was brought to hospital where she was observed by Levy. She was referred to an off-reservation hospital in May 1963.

Two years and four months had elapsed since she was first hospitalized. Her behavior during this period was marked by heavy drinking and some promiscuity. In 1960, the smoking ritual from Mountainway was performed. Datura, one of the Frenzy-witchcraftway medicines, was also administered at this ceremony. An Enemyway was performed after she had seen men fighting, and a Nightway was recommended but never performed because, while at a peyote meeting, she had cried out like a *yei*. She was said to be *diitła*. A Windway and a Shootingway were also tried but to no effect.

The family and the leader of the peyote meetings Mildred attended confirmed the fact that her catatonic states had been preceded by the ingestion of peyote. The peyote leader told us that sometimes she seemed better at a peyote meeting but that, at other times, her condition worsened. The family mentioned that she had fainted after taking datura during one of the Frenzy-witchcraftway ceremonies. During her second hospital stay, psychiatrists found no evidence of psychosis. Nor were any other pathological symptoms noted. She was sent home after being advised not to eat peyote, and she has not become catatonic since.

Mildred remarried in 1963 and resumed her hand-trembling practice. She also learned the sucking cure, although she did not perform the Suckingway ceremonial. Her parents felt that she had been cured, and it is possible that by sucking and hand trembling she was channeling her propensity for conversion reactions. Yet, when seen by Gutmann in 1964, she was constantly sucking and gnawing on her fingers, especially during the administration of the Thematic Apperception Test. Gutmann found nothing to suggest the withdrawal and autism of schizophrenia. Her responses to the TAT included stories of children who defied their parents, of birds that flew into fires, and of whirlwinds. She also told stories of children grieving because their mother abandoned them but who were defiant and mastered the trauma by actively inviting and provoking the loss of love. Gutmann's impression was that she "goes to excess in action, thought and fantasy and is not concerned with the consequences. A willful woman who gives evidence that defiance and externalization fends off experiences of emptiness and loss."

Two years after our interviews, in 1966, we were able to get an Indian Health Service psychiatrist to interview Mildred in her home. It appears that not all had gone well after her second hospitalization. During 1964 and 1965 she had been delusional. In particular, she was afraid that her second husband was trying to poison her and, on one occasion, she asked her parents for a gun so that she could shoot him. This incident convinced them that something more had to be done, and another hand trembler was consulted.

During the ritual, she felt that she was on the right track at last; "A weight began to lift from my mind." She was told that her only hope was to have a Frenzy-witchcraftway performed by a particular singer who lived some distance from her home. This ceremonialist was difficult to find and, when located, told them that the whole family was involved and they all must take part. He insisted further that the sing must be performed at his home and not theirs. Mildred and her parents were so impressed by the hand trembler and the singer that they followed advice and had the ceremony performed. Datura was administered, but this time the results were beneficial. Mildred felt that the singer was very powerful and that he "was praying my thoughts back into my mind." By the end of the ceremony, she felt that she had completely recovered.

Throughout this interview, Mildred, who was neatly dressed, related appropriately and affectionately to all members of her family while industriously spinning wool. She was friendly and quite frank about her illness. She demonstrated considerable range of affect appropriate to the story she was telling, speaking fluently and coherently. The psychiatrist's impression was that there had been a complete remission of her schizophrenic reaction, which was apparently of mixed type. He also felt that the Frenzy-witchcraftway and the datura were instrumental in effecting the cure.

In actuality, however, things did not improve as much as had been hoped. Even after the Frenzy-witchcraftway she would have spells of dizziness, loss of consciousness, and several hours of weakness whenever she performed the hand-trembling ritual. She was paid for her service in jewelry and became anxious about who would care for her wealth when she "was gone." She was also worried about getting her jewelry out of pawn when the payments came due.

Between 1965 and 1975 she gave birth to five children by her second husband. She complained of lower back pain and was frequently depressed and plagued by nightmares. She was concerned about her husband's drinking and her children's well-being. In defiance of her parents' wishes, she and her husband continued to attend peyote meetings and her husband stopped drinking. The turning point came, finally, in 1971 when, at the age of thirty-five, she found the courage and sense of independence to defy her family and to reject hand trembling entirely. The security provided by her second marriage and participation in the peyote religion which helped her husband to stop drinking made this newly found independence possible.

When we last spoke to her, in 1975, she and her husband were living away from her parents in Tuba City in a neat, well-cared-for house with a modern kitchen and well-tended yard and garden. Despite the fact that she was found to have a lumbar degenerative disease the year before, she felt that her major troubles were over and that her life was finally her own. After discussing similar problems encountered by her cousin, she offered the opinion that only well people should become hand tremblers. She was sad that her family could never understand this and felt that many of her problems could have been avoided if she had not been forced to become a hand trembler.

Alice was five years older than her cousin Mildred and led a life that paralleled hers in many respects. Their fathers and another brother were singers as well as diagnosticians. None of the sons became ceremonialists because, it was said, they drank too much. But each man had a daughter who was prevailed upon to become a hand trembler. The family's hopes were disappointed in Alice's and Mildred's cases but the daughter of the youngest brother became a well-known and successful diagnostician at the same time that she was educated and held a well-paying job in the federal school system. This was in contrast to Alice and Mildred, neither of whom could speak English.

In 1954, when she was twenty-three years of age, Alice's parents died within a short time of each other. Then, four years later while she was in a tuberculosis sanitorium, her first husband died in an automobile accident. Early in 1961 she had an ectopic pregnancy, and it was shortly thereafter that she experienced her first seizure and was first diagnosed by a hand trembler. In this year also she began to keep company with a young man ten years younger than she, who was to become her second husband. We recall that, after her return from the sanitorium, she began to see a lot of her cousin Mildred, who was also having problems. The two years from 1961 to 1963 were marked by marital discord and seizures and terminated by the dissolution of the second marriage and her hospitalization. Although her family says that she was brought to hospital for her seizures on several occasions, her medical chart indicates that she never complained of them. She had violent quarrels with her husband, and in at least one instance he beat her. Her husband resented that he was expected to live with her son by her first husband who, at eighteen, was only four years his junior. He felt that his bad behavior was caused by Alice who, he said, was trying to witch him. The family believed that the marital discord and the final separation of the couple were the cause of Alice's seizures.

Two seizures, which conformed to descriptions obtained from the family, were seen in hospital in 1963, when Alice was thirty-two years old. She would lie down on the floor, neither moving nor responding. Sometimes she would call out her dead parents' names and say that they were coming for her and that she was going away with them. At other times she would lie quietly, breathing slowly. She appeared to be awake but did not respond to painful stimuli. After a short time, she would abruptly regain consciousness and talk freely. The physical exam was negative. On the second day of her hospital stay, she had a seizure that involved some slight trembling of the left hand. She never ran off or tore at her clothing. There was no foaming at the mouth, cyanosis, or thrashing about. The seizures were considered hysterical, and she was referred to an off-reservation hospital, where her EEG was normal and the psychiatrist confirmed the impression of conversion reaction.

When diagnosed by hand trembling in 1961, her trouble was said to have been caused by the ghost of her dead infant. For this the blackening ritual of Evilway was performed. No diagnoses were made after this, and no other ceremonies were performed. Presumably this was because her parents were dead and her uncles did not take the same interest in her that they did in their own children.

When interviewed by Gutmann and Parker in 1964, Alice "was surly, resentful, and uncooperative although she did give responses to the Thematic Apperception Test. She was argumentative, displayed some paranoid features, and demanded that Parker make restitution for damage done to her truck windows by guests at an Enemyway sponsored by his parents some years before."

Her TAT responses were "atypical for people complaining of ghost contamination as well as for others generally in that the main affect overtly expressed is aggression. This aggression is between people who try to wrest things from each other and, in a more impersonal fashion, between cars about to collide. There is much evidence that she handles the more dysphoric, deprived, and empty feelings through externalization and somatization. In cards where others typically experience sadness and isolation, she sees people falling asleep and being blind. These are both forms of somatically expressed denial. She also sees snow, suggesting dissociated experiences of depression."

"Impression: I see her along lines of anaclitic paranoia; a woman who projects strong oral aggressive feelings onto others and, then, is free to fight them for the 'goodies,' the targets of her aggression now identified as the 'selfish' ones. She probably stresses aggression and somatization as a way of avoiding strong feelings of deprivation engendered by the loss of her parents, Child, and both husbands. In effect, all affects and difficulties are externalized as malign influences rather than inner pain, hunger, or emptiness."

From the time of our interviews until 1971 when she was forty years old, Alice continued to have numerous hysterical seizures similar to those already described. She drank heavily and fought frequently with her neighbors and her son. She was also involved in two automobile accidents but escaped without suffering serious injury. Alice married for the third time in 1971 and, by the end of the year, her symptoms changed radically. On three occasions she was admitted to hospital suffering from speech loss and a choking sensation which was diagnosed as globus hystericus, a conversion reaction. These episodes lasted as long as two hours. She feared she was being witched and complained that her family was unsympathetic. She visited the mental health clinic frequently and became very dependent on Valium, a tranquilizer. After being married only a few months, her husband left her for another woman. She was soon seen in hospital in a suicidal state, complaining that her husband was trying to kill her with birth control pills.

The family, who up to this time felt that Alice's drinking would interfere with a hand-trembling career, changed their minds after Mildred refused to work at it any longer and prevailed upon her to have the Hand-tremblingway performed. We recall that on some occasions, at least, her seizure episodes included some slight trembling in one arm. For a brief time she was successful and gained some renown in the community when, in a trance, she followed a ball of fire only she could see to the spot where some stolen jewelry had been hidden. Some twenty to thirty people were in attendance, following her for several miles. Witnesses maintain that the jewelry was in fact found. Immediately, she was in great demand as a diagnostician and seer, and was paid quite well for her services, usually with jewelry. Soon, however, she became anxiety ridden about her wealth and would pawn items of jewelry at several trading posts. Then, when she failed to redeem them, the pawned items would be put up for sale and she would have a hysterical attack.

A year later, after the spells of speechlessness, she fainted while herding sheep. She blamed all these problems on the hand trembling. She complained of dizziness, loss of consciousness, and headaches, until finally she asked the hospital mental health staff to give her a signed statement testifying that hand trembling was bad for her health. It was not clear whether she wanted this letter to convince her family or her clients. For the remainder of 1972, she was seen several times for insomnia and chest pains. On one occasion she was depressed and talked about suicide. Alice stopped hand trembling in 1973. She still came to hospital frequently for tranquilizers but always claimed she was too rushed to talk over her problems. In 1974 she had another spell of dizziness and blacking out and another episode of globus hystericus. Throughout 1975 she was seen in the mental health clinic every month and became quite dependent on her medications but, aside from anxiety, she had few complaints.

Discussion

Between 50 and 70 percent of singers in various parts of the reservation learned their ceremonies from their fathers, brothers, maternal uncles, or maternal grandfathers (Henderson 1982). Singers often marry herbalists or hand tremblers. Their sons become singers and the daughters herbalists or diagnosticians. The desire to keep ceremonial knowledge in the family was the overriding reason for Mildred and Alice to become diagnosticians.

Both these young women experienced episodes of hand trembling prior to being initiated. But the "gift" may be transmitted in a more mechanical manner, as the story of Parker's brother, chosen to inherit from his stepfather, illustrates. While camping one night on a journey, the older man began to hand-tremble and to repeatedly slap the younger man's arm, thus transmitting the power by contact. The visible sign of success came when the youth's arm began to tremble. It is interesting that none of the individuals who spontaneously produced the required trembling or shaking in one arm and who were not from a family of a hand trembler were ever said to qualify. This does not rule out the possibility that such cases do exist; none, however, came to our attention. We can only speculate on what might have happened in Carl's case if his family had not been so unsympathetic to his religious aspirations. Certainly Mary's father was a singer and could have arranged for her to be initiated, but he had already begun to suspect that some of his daughter's attacks were self-willed.

Neither Alice nor Mildred were cured when they became hand tremblers. Instead, performing the ritual exacerbated their symptoms. It is our guess that Clarissa also had personal problems which may have led her to become a hand trembler and, subsequently, to relinquish the role. It is certain that she continued to have hysterical attacks for the rest of her adult life.

Because this study has focused on seizures and is not a survey of practicing hand tremblers, we cannot say that no hand trembler has had his or her hysterical symptoms eased by practicing this form of diagnosis. Clarissa, we recall, came to medical attention only because she was in hospital with tuberculosis. It is, then, possible that individuals with histrionic personalities or mild conversion hysterias might perform their professional tasks adequately and, at the same time, have their symptoms made bearable if not cured entirely. At this time, however, we can only say that none of the successfully practicing hand tremblers known to us appears in any way abnormal and none of the performances we have seen looked at all like hysterical episodes.

The three women who did become hand tremblers exhibited the appropriate signs—the shaking or trembling in one arm only. That this behavior is learned is suggested by the fact that none of these were epileptic seizures. We did find a tendency for some people to be influenced by cultural expectations and to present bilateral trembling as if it were unilateral, often by holding one extremity with the other. We can only speculate whether such cases are ever taken to be signs of the gift for hand trembling. Similarly, we cannot tell whether the epileptics with simple partial seizures involving only one side of the body were not thought to be hand tremblers because their convulsions were not restricted to the extremity but involved the whole side of the body, because the affliction was too debilitating, or because none of them came from families of hand tremblers. Without an extensive study of hand tremblers and a control group for comparison, we can only suggest that Navajo hand tremblers (a) may be normal or neurotic but probably not psychotic or epileptic; (b) the mildly neurotic may be cured or helped but the more severe hysterics cannot succeed in the role; (c) there may be several routes to hand-trembler status but inheritance is probably the most common.

CHAPTER 7

Frenzy Witchcraft

The signs of frenzy witchcraft are more varied than those of hand trembling, which are confined to motion of one extremity only. Typically, the victim may utter a brief cry, run about aimlessly or in circles, tear at her clothing, and disappear into the night. Physicians would consider such episodes to be dissociative states or, possibly, complex partial seizures. Dissociative states are characterized by an altered state of consciousness, the retention of more or less full control of motor and sensory systems, and amnesia for the episode. Navajos tend to label such spells of behavior as frenzy witchcraft without insisting on the presence of each and every element. There are indications that a fairly wide range of conditions might be labeled as frenzy witchcraft. A woman suffering from hypothyroidism, identified in the community survey as having "spells," had Frenzy-witchcraftway performed because, at times, her attacks involved yelling and running around the hospital ward.

Six epileptics and six hysterics experienced either complex partial seizures or conversion reactions that emulated them, either alone or in combination with other kinds of seizures. Four of these will not be examined. Two were epileptics who combined generalized epileptic seizures with hysterical fugue states and who had committed incest. These cases will be discussed in some detail in the following chapter. Clarissa, we have seen, had been a hand trembler. Her persistent bouts of uncontrolled hand trembling indicated that her problem derived from the mismanagement of this power. Her dissociative states were infrequent and were seen as complications of the hand-trembling disorder. Alice, we recall, was an orphan whose relatives were not disposed to arrange for ceremonial treatments until she was chosen to become a hand trembler in Mildred's place. Among the eight cases we shall examine here,

only one was not given a diagnosis specifically denoting seizures. Two were diagnosed as suffering from Coyote-caused disorders, two from frenzy witchcraft, and three from both causes.

Belinda was a young woman with a cleft palate. Why she was
not diagnosed when her hysterical seizures started is not entirely clear. She was brought to hospital by her family because
of spells during which she pulled her hair, screamed, sometimes ran off, saw vague shapes coming after her, and for which
she had retrograde amnesia. Her parents kept her out of school
until she was thirteen years old because they wished to protect
her from the outside world. When she was finally forced to go
to school, she was never able to keep up with her classmates
because she was constantly undergoing operations for her cleft
palate. It seems also that she was teased because of her defor-
mity. Finally, she and her parents developed a very negative attitude toward the multistage operations required to correct the
cleft palate, which were still not completed and which had not
corrected her speech defect. She was removed from school and
remained at home until she began to have spells of dissociative
behavior and was brought to hospital. At this juncture, she was
sent to an off-reservation mental hospital for evaluation and an
effort was made to speed up the course of her corrective surgery. She was, by this time, twenty-one years of age.

Belinda denied ever having the attacks described by her parents which, according to them, occurred at night. Occasionally
an attack would be preceded by her seeing tall figures trying to
touch her. Then she would either fall down unconscious or
have convulsions, during which her body would jerk intermit-
tently, her fists would clench, and she would pull her hair. No
physician had been able to observe one of her seizures. At the
conclusion of a three-week stay in a mental hospital, the psychiatric report noted that there was no evidence of neurological
or psychiatric disease. "It must be emphasized, however, that
while superficial contact was good, there was never any real
rapport. Patient did not feel she could communicate. Since we
have observed nothing that would be called grossly abnormal
except for some degree of emotional flattening, some reticence,

and some intellectual deficit of minor nature, the only diagnosis that could be made now from her history would be one of conversion hysteria."

To us the parents confided that an Enemy-Monsterway had been performed for her cleft palate when she was only two years old. The diagnosis involved prenatal influence, but the parents were reluctant to reveal the exact causal factor. Although an early history of spells was denied to hospital personnel, to us the parents said that she had had spells as a child for which the blackening ritual from Evilway was performed and, later, a two-night form of the Lifeway. These ceremonies, they claimed, had "fixed her up," and there had been no recurrence of spells until she was twenty years old.

Belinda married when she was twenty-five and bore two children. The first had a cleft palate; the second was premature and died at twenty-one months of age. She became depressed and made a mild suicide gesture. Two years later, however, she gave birth to a normal child, and two more normal births followed. She was pregnant with her sixth child in 1975, when she was thirty-three years of age. She appeared to be in good health and happy in her marriage.

We suspect the parents were embarrassed by the presence of a seizure condition caused by a prenatal influence and wanted to avoid the stigma of seizure-specific ceremonies. Had there been no cleft palate, it might have been easier to accept a diagnosis of frenzy witchcraft which would lay the blame at some distance from the parents' door. Congenital deformities are thought to be evidence of a father's witchcraft.

Laura was diagnosed early in life by a hand trembler, who said that her father had killed a rabid dog while her mother was pregnant. Laura's mother was said to have died from *yistezh*, a sexual infection of the genitals caused by Coyote contamination. In consequence, the family has attempted to avoid stigmatization and has never had any Coyote ritual performed for her. They have, however, had a Lifeway performed for the chronicity of her problem, as well as a Shootingway and a Chiricahua Windway for other etiologies. In addition to her epileptic major seizures, there were some episodes of bizarre be-havior that once involved baring her breasts in public and some episodes of violence.

Another patient, a thirty-year-old married woman whose conversion symptoms began with a month of daily fainting spells preceded by some senseless speech, was thought to be suffering from witchcraft and was treated by a Hopi healer who "sucked some stones out of her." She was subsequently treated with a Windway. A hand trembler then diagnosed lightning contamination and a Shootingway was performed. Finally, some form of Coyoteway was performed. The family, unfortunately, was unwilling to talk about the diagnosis.

Turning now to those who were treated with Frenzy-witchcraftway, we find, first, that the expected stories of sexual witchcraft are conspicuous by their absence; second, that Coyote is diagnosed as a cause of the symptoms as often as frenzy witchcraft; and, finally, that violence and paranoid delusions are featured in many of the seizure episodes. Mildred and her parents, it will be recalled, thought that the family of the "other" woman was working frenzy witchcraft against her. This sounds more like witchery, the major form of Navajo witchcraft, because neither Mildred nor her errant husband appear to have been seduced by love magic. Indeed, sexual excess is not prominently featured in any of the accounts provided us, although there was a period during which she drank and had some casual liaisons. Mildred saw scenes of violence, believed both her husbands were trying to kill her, and had outbursts of violence. Frenzy-witchcraftway was performed on two separate occasions but so was the smoking ritual from the Mountainway which pertains to the evil of Coyote and his Bear wife. We recall also that Carl was thought to be suffering from frenzy witchcraft. His uncle was said to be the witch, who, having already killed the father, was now trying to kill Carl. Carl lived in the Fort Defiance Service Unit where Frenzy-witchcraftway is extinct. In consequence, he was treated with the Turning Basket ritual. Susan, another epileptic living in the Fort Defiance area, was treated with Gameway, which is considered a branch of Frenzy-witchcraftway (Luckert 1978:3–6).

Susan was orphaned at the age of two and adopted by her childless aunt and uncle. She had generalized epileptic seizures which began when she was thirteen years old and which were well controlled by antiepileptic medication. Three years later she began to have attacks of bizarre behavior which, when seen by physicians, were thought to be hysterical. One of these episodes was described by her mother: "Soon a woman outside saw her fall down. We had a hard time trying to get her inside. She was angry and she was kicking and hitting at us. She would try to bite when we picked her up and we had to tie her legs." Whenever her husband did anything that displeased her, she would respond with these bizarre bouts of anger during which she often saw her deceased parents and uncle. Her first major sing was Mountainway. Later, after having a Male and Female Shootingway, the Gameway was performed. A Turning Basket ritual was also performed and, later, the smoking ritual from the Mountainway. The diagnosed etiologies were always innocuous. According to her aunt, the first Mountainway was given because she saw bears while in hospital and Susan believed she was given bear meat while away at school. The family believed she needed Gameway after a Hopi crystal gazer told them she had been contaminated by a deer. Although Susan's epileptic seizures began when she was thirteen years old, the hysterical episodes had their start after the death of the uncle who had adopted her. She maintains that she was very fond of him because "he always brought me presents." Her first husband deserted her soon after their marriage, and her relationship with the second is stormy.

Elizabeth had hysterical seizures which the family thought were due to the witchcraft of her father. In this instance also the witch was seeking to harm the family he had deserted, and the account sounds more like witchery. Yet Elizabeth was diagnosed as suffering from frenzy witchcraft and, in addition to Frenzy-witchcraftway, the Turning Basket ritual and the smoking ceremony from Gameway were performed. We believe that the seizures determined the diagnoses, despite the fact that the supposed witchcraft did not resemble sexual magic. The psychological dynamics of the case are compatible, however, with psychiatric notions about the genesis of hysteria in young women.

In 1964, Elizabeth was thirty-one years old, married, and with several children. She spoke about having to overcome the sullen resistance of her father in order to go to school and obtain an eighth-grade education. She believed that her parents wanted to keep her poor. After completing school and getting married, she and her husband settled in a large city on the northwest coast. Their economic success and happiness were a personal triumph for the couple, who believed they would never return to the reservation. Her seizures began suddenly without recognizable cause. Episodes of severe frontal headaches were followed by hours of semiconscious behavior. "I was talking to myself and asking for my mother. I was that way for three hours." At the hospital, physicians were unable to find any organic cause for these symptoms.

A telephone call to her mother at home complicated the situation. She was urged to return home with the children. On her arrival, she was informed that she was not the only one in the family who was ill. Her mother believed that Elizabeth's father, who had left her mother and remarried, was now witching her and all the children. None of the other members of the family had experienced seizures, however, and all were in good health in 1964.

Elizabeth remained with her mother for the next year and became increasingly involved in attempts to counteract her father's witchcraft. With each new discovery of how her father was trying to destroy them, her symptoms proliferated. During an Evilway, she had a spell in which her hands were clenched, her legs pulled up, and she saw men. "They stood around me and said 'come along with us.' They were my father's friends." At this time she also began to have chest pains. A hand trembler said that her father had taken some of her hair or fingernail parings and put them under a datura plant, thus necessitating the Frenzy-witchcraftway. They were also told that her father had placed an automobile part that had been in contact with datura by the road at a dangerous spot to cause a car accident.

She gained employment at the hospital but never complained about her symptoms, believing that the white doctors would not be able to help her kind of trouble. When her husband finally returned to the reservation, he was surprised and chagrined to discover he was expected to stay and help pay for the ceremonies. Some malicious gossip about his wife initiated a series of jealous arguments. For a year and a half, from 1960 to 1961, the couple stayed together arguing about whether they should really stay on the reservation. The husband continued to resent the financial burden imposed on him by the number of sings being performed.

In 1961 the husband lost control of himself and beat Elizabeth and her mother so that they sustained lacerations and were brought to hospital. Five days later, she became confused and semiconscious for two hours and had to be restrained so that she would not run off. Four days after this episode, she complained of headaches at work and that night was admitted to hospital in a confused, semiconscious state. The attendant physicians believed her spell was a conversion reaction and referred her to an off-reservation hospital for evaluation, where a neurological exam and an EEG were normal.

Elizabeth experienced no further seizures after her return from the hospital. Nevertheless, seven more ceremonies were performed during the following year. The family wanted to make sure she was "really well," and Elizabeth feels that the sings were worthwhile because witches tend to leave their victims alone once they have made them poor; the family had certainly been impoverished by the number of sings they paid for. They lost their truck and were behind on bills but intended to continue with ceremonial treatments as soon as they were able. Opposed to this rather negative and unusual estimation of the success of ceremonial cures was the belief that the ceremonials did, in fact, turn the witchcraft back on its perpetrators. "Some of my father's friends have died since then but my dad and two others are still living. I wish my dad would die. I just can't stand to see him around. He tries to be so friendly whenever I see him."

Elizabeth's responses to the Thematic Apperception Test highlighted stories of resentment of her mother's control over her, of being old and sad, and of fast, dangerous driving. It looks as if she was able to express resentment against her father after he had left the family and she could blame all her symptoms on him but that her feelings about her mother were still difficult to express openly. She and her husband remained on the reservation; when we again contacted her in 1975, she had experienced no recurrence of her psychiatric symptoms.

Mary's generalized epileptic seizures were overlaid by hysterical fugue states and one episode of hand trembling. In 1964, she was seventeen years of age, the oldest of five children. Her father was a Chiricahua Windway singer and a heavy drinker who had been arrested on numerous occasions for drunkenness and bootlegging. As a child he had suffered from fecal incontinence until the age of twelve. When we knew the family, their major source of support was social welfare.

At school Mary had the reputation of being willful and pampered. She had stolen from her classmates, cut classes, worn too much makeup, and threatened suicide when punished. A twelve-year-old younger brother who was retarded and had frequent major seizures was, for some reason, her favorite sibling. There were also, in 1964, two younger sisters and a baby brother who were all normal. Their mother appeared very subdued and retiring.

After some poorly described bouts of unconsciousness when she was two years old, Mary was seizure free until she was fourteen, when she experienced an episode of hysterical paraplegia, or paralysis of both legs. This condition was cured after two visits to a Hopi healer, who "sucked" an eagle talon from her groin. When she was fifteen, her grandfather died and her younger brother was institutionalized. These events were followed by two years of frequent seizures which went untreated for some months. Several episodes began with the announcement that an unidentified man was trying to get her: "I don't know him. It's like his face was covered with wool—something like a medicine man but nothing special." After experiencing this aura, she would run in circles before falling to the ground thrashing about wildly. She would then recover with retrograde amnesia. One day at school, she suddenly began hitting a well-liked teacher, after which she fell to the floor thrashing about.

This attack led to her admission to hospital, where she was found unconscious on the floor after having gone to the bathroom. Her only complaint at that time was some abdominal pain. She groaned continuously, thrashed about, and resisted examination. Only the arrival of her father who spoke to her in Navajo made her start to respond. She became more alert before lapsing into sleep. After this she would stare into space and could not respond to questioning. Later she admitted to a fear of epilepsy because of her brother.

She was transferred to a mental hospital for evaluation where, although her EEG was generally within normal limits, there was a burst of high-voltage, unilateral theta activity. The duration of this burst was less than half a second, but superimposed were some fast components that gave the discharge a rather sharp form. About ten seconds later, an isolated sharp discharge arose in the left frontotemporal region. The EEG was not repeated. Two nights before she was discharged from hospital, she was heard to cry out and a nurse found her thrashing about in bed complaining of severe chest and abdominal pain. A physical examination was completely negative. It was then learned that another Indian girl in the same room had approached her sexually and that this had precipitated the attack. Within a few hours she had quieted down and become her "old, happy self." She was returned to the reservation with the diagnosis of "psychoneurosis, much improved."

After her return home a hand trembler made two diagnoses. The first was that Mary's father had been contaminated by a rabid dog during her mother's pregnancy. For this a one-night fumigation ritual from the Mountainway was performed. The second diagnosis was that someone was working frenzy witchcraft against her. A Frenzy-witchcraftway was begun, but halfway through the proceedings she had a spell in which voices told her that if she completed the ceremonial she would be dead within three days and that she should go to the Mormons to have prayers said over her instead. These proved ineffectual, and another visit to the Hopi healer revealed that to really destroy the witch would be beyond the financial means of the family.

At this juncture, Mary initiated a new direction in therapy.

She began to dream of her dead grandfather instead of the unidentified man. He told her to have Navajo ceremonies performed or she would die. When she had these spells, she would see her grandfather sitting in the corner looking as he had before he died. Another hand trembler said that she was being disturbed by the grandfather's ghost and by that of a girl who lived nearby and who had died not long before. An Evilway ceremony was performed, but the spells continued unabated. Mary threw tantrums and bit members of the family. In despair they brought her to the hospital so that she could be sent away for another evaluation. Once there, however, she changed her mind about leaving the reservation and, after an hour, left against medical advice. The moment she returned home she began to diagnose her own condition by hand trembling as described in the preceding chapter, although she knew none of the prerequisite prayers. Her spells continued over the succeeding months, and, on one occasion after behaving strangely throughout the evening, she bolted out of the house during the night. Her father followed and found her thrashing about on her back. She was laughing—and gasped out something about people coming after her. Again, she was only calmed by her father holding her. Following this episode, Whirling Coyote prayers from the Mountainway were performed for the earlier diagnosis of rabid dog contamination.

Later Mary married a boy she had been seeing for some time, although he was aware of her illness. The couple went to live in Utah, where she was seizure free for a year. They returned home when she had another seizure. After her return she had about two seizures each month. She would get abdominal pain, fall down, and get "real tight." Her mouth would clench, but she did not thrash about as she had in her earlier spells. She was not cyanotic, did not become incontinent, and did not bite her tongue. Then a second Frenzy-witchcraftway was performed, this time without interruption, and she remained seizure free for five years. The marriage remained intact and children were born in 1965 and 1967.

By 1969 the marriage had deteriorated markedly. The husband appeared normal, but he drank frequently and ran after other women. Mary began to complain of chest pains and would occasionally scream and become unresponsive. Within the year, the marriage disintegrated and Mary took to drinking and having affairs with a number of men. One of her younger sisters, now eighteen years old, began to have hysterical symptoms at this time also. During 1970, she continued to drink, engaged in promiscuous behavior, and experienced chest pains and anxiety attacks. On one occasion, depressed and suicidal, she decided to take Antabuse in an effort to control her drinking.

The following year, at age twenty-four, she gave birth to an illegitimate child by Caesarean section. In 1972, after a drunken fight with a boyfriend, she attempted suicide with an overdose of Antabuse and Darvon and was admitted to hospital in a comatose state. There she was diagnosed as having an underlying schizophrenic personality with depressive and hysterical features. Two months later, she underwent an operation for chronic cholecystitis and a tubo-ovarian abscess. Only a few weeks later, she was in an automobile accident and, while in the X-ray room, suffered a major generalized seizure which the attendant physician said was epileptic. A second suicide attempt by drug overdose followed the accident by two weeks.

During 1973, Mary continued drinking while living with her family. After a four-day binge, she began to tremble while in her father's bedroom and to have palpitations followed by general weakness. Two months later, she was admitted to the hospital for a hysterical seizure which involved stiffening of the extremities and clenched fists followed by several hours of unresponsiveness. She stopped taking antiepileptic medication in 1974 and subsequently had a major generalized seizure at home during a thunderstorm. On admission, she was observed to be in a postictal stupor. The description given by the family was detailed, and the physician felt confident in pronouncing it epileptic.

That same year, Mary went to live in a nearby border town. In 1975, she was working as a barmaid in a bar with a large Indian clientele, still drinking and feeling depressed generally. One of her sisters was killed in an automobile accident that year, and Mary felt she could never live with her parents again.

She was taking her medication regularly and had been seizure
free during the first half of the year. Her parents continued to
care for her children.

Gutmann interviewed her and administered a Thematic Apperception Test in 1964. He felt she had "a rather tart, ob-
viously close, eroticized relationship with her father who was
present (she darted glances at him and shared 'in' jokes)." She
was actively mourning her grandfather and has felt 'empty inside' since he died. She also missed her brother who was institutionalized in Phoenix."

Her TAT responses included "atypical stories of interpersonal aggression, defiance of parents, and deprivation, isolation, and hunger as the seeming punishment for this." His
impression was of "a rather aggressive, independent girl who is
afraid of the consequences of independence and sexual maturity. There is an Oedipal involvement with her father which
probably heightens her need to cling to parental modes. He is
probably the faceless man who comes after her. She covers his
face because she cannot give expression to her erotic feelings
toward him. . . . Her Oedipal feelings are experienced as an externalized assault by their object, her father."

Discussion

Psychologically these cases of dissociation have a common
theme: rebellion against the father and the ambivalence generated by this defiance. Anger, aggression, anxiety, and depression are all present. Hysterical fits partly represent a rage
reaction due to frustration of genital sexual wishes. Mary's
erotic involvement with her father is clear, as is her need to
free herself from it and her fear of the consequences. The other
women we have described seek to free themselves from domineering fathers who force them to become hand tremblers or
thwart desires to leave home to attend school. Whether further
investigation of these cases would clarify underlying sexual
conflicts must remain moot. Here our concern is with the relationship of the diagnoses to the seizures.

Eight people with hysterical dissociative states were diagnosed and, with one exception, treated. A Coyote etiology was

identified as often as frenzy witchcraft (frenzy witchcraft, 2; frenzy witchcraft *and* Coyote, 3; Coyote, 2; other, 1). This can not have come about because Frenzy-witchcraftway is almost extinct. Not only were we able to locate ten singers in the Tuba City area who performed this ceremony, but Gameway is an acceptable substitute. Moreover, singers of Coyoteway and other Coyote rituals are equally rare. Even when frenzy witchcraft was diagnosed, however, the accounts given us told of witchery rather than of love magic, and the father was either identified as the witch or was the source of personal conflict.

Carl was thought to be witched by an uncle who wished to kill both the father and the son. Carl's hysterical fits began immediately after his father died and were accompanied by attempts to identify himself with a singer who had been his father's friend. We can only speculate whether Carl's psychological problems resulted from an unresolved Oedipal conflict that produced feelings of guilt when his father died and that he tried to assuage by identifying with a father surrogate. Like Carl, Susan's bouts of hysteria started after the death of her uncle who adopted her when she was two years old. Although we know little of their relationship, she saw him during her fits, claimed that he indulged her, and had two difficult marriages.

Elizabeth believed that her father was trying to cause her death with datura. Her psychological problems centered on her resentment of both her father and mother. The woman who experienced fainting spells also complained that her parents kept her at home to herd sheep and would not let her go away to school, although she wanted very much to do so. A Hopi healer said she was being witched, and ultimately some form of Coyoteway was performed. We were not told whether a particular person had come under suspicion.

Mary, whose father was a singer, could not identify the person who came after her and who, she said, was "something like a medicine man, nothing special." Mary was never told who was witching her or why, but her eroticised feelings for her father were clearly the source of her anxiety. Although Mildred and her family believed that the "other woman" was trying to destroy her, it was clear that her illness was an expression of her ambivalent feelings toward her father who attempted to control her.

From our point of view, these patients have more than their seizures in common. For most, we think the father is the source of psychological conflict. How they are perceived by Navajos, however, is more difficult to ascertain. Why, we want to know, was frenzy witchcraft diagnosed when the stories were so clearly those of witchery calling for an Evilway cure? Is it that the form of the seizure is so firmly identified with love magic that the diagnosis and treatment follows automatically? Or does the tendency also to diagnose a Coyote etiology indicate that, recognizing a larger community of seizures, the diagnosticians and singers are connecting these dissociative states with the incest of Coyote and his daughters? Although the answers to these questions cannot be attempted here, they will be discussed in the final chapter, after the cases of moth madness are described.

CHAPTER 8

Moth Madness

Moth madness, like AIDS (autoimmune deficiency syndrome) in contemporary American society, is the dread disease of the Navajos. The appearance of the fearful signs of the major motor seizure make it clear to all that the epileptic has committed incest with a sibling or clan relative. Even if the onset is in the first few years of life, it is believed that one of the parents has transgressed a tabu and the disease has been transmitted to the child by prenatal contact. It seemed unlikely that hysterics would have much to gain by emulating major motor seizures, but it was not at all clear how epileptics and their families would avoid the stigma.

We have already seen that nine of the ten epileptics with major seizures who sought ceremonial cures were treated with the Coyote rituals, which today serve as substitutes for the extinct Mothway. This suggests that the many alternate diagnoses possible in the Navajo scheme of causation are not adequate protection in the event seizures persist. The practice of isolating defective children to protect the child and the family from a hostile environment has also been mentioned. This chapter will look at the lives of the hysterics and the epileptics with generalized seizures to determine how the hysterics escape the dreaded diagnosis and whether the epileptics' difficult lives are caused by society or by the disease itself.

The Hysterics

Although there were six hysterics whose spells were assigned to the generalized seizure category, two had only a single episode. Another's fugue states were dramatic and attracted more attention, so that she was more like a victim of frenzy witchcraft. The symptoms of two others were variable and did not look much like convulsions. One, a young woman, had bouts of trembling in both arms. As she was very acculturated and spoke no Navajo, she was never diagnosed by hand tremblers or her family. Another woman experienced minor tremors which started in both arms but soon involved her whole body at the same time that her skin broke out in a red rash. These symptoms were infrequent and were not perceived as salient, so that she was treated with sings not specifically for seizures. There was only one hysteric who had spells that looked like major seizures.

Carla was forty-six years old, in 1964, a widow with nine children who had a one-year history of seizure-like behavior. She was uneducated, spoke no English, and had led a life characterized by deprivation and loss. When she was quite young, her father deserted her mother and she was sent to live with a busy grandmother who gave her little attention. Life became somewhat brighter after her mother remarried; she went home again to find that her stepfather was kind and attentive.

When she was eleven years old, a brother-in-law murdered her sister and her stepfather. Years later, she married a man who was a good provider. Together they had eight children. With most of the children grown, the couple entered middle life. Then the husband, after being arrested for bootlegging, went into a coma, had convulsions, and died while Carla was taking him home. Following this shock, she was asked to view her husband's brain, which had been placed in a jar after the autopsy so that the physician could explain to her what had caused his sudden demise. This experience, she told us, was most unnerving. Levy had seen the brain earlier and had remonstrated with the physician, explaining about the Navajos' fear of ghost contamination, but to no avail.

For a year, Carla carried on with her life, as there were still some children at home. Soon, however, she was pregnant and began to get pains in her chest from doing heavy chores. She would dream that her husband came to her asking that she keep the children at home to care for them, that, in effect, she give them the care her mother was unable to give her when she was a child. Despite her efforts, however, she was soon forced to give the younger children into the care of others.

Then news came that her son-in-law had been killed in an automobile accident. At the funeral her chest pains became acute and, a few weeks later, she was admitted to hospital in an unconscious state. On the morning of admission, she had fallen to the ground and had begun to shake all over. The shaking continued for two hours, until she was brought to the hospital by a visiting social worker. There she was observed to make writhing movements. Initially, she would not communicate. The neurological exam was normal, and the writhing stopped within fifteen minutes. For the next twelve months she had many bouts of chest pain and dizziness followed by an hour or two of unconsciousness. She was given tranquilizers and felt that they helped more than some of the sings that had been performed for her.

The stressful events that preceded her initial attack pointed to ghost contamination. For this condition, a blackening and a reddening ritual from Evilway was performed, as well as a Shootingway and a prayer ceremony (ákéké sóódizon). But, as her attacks did not last for more than one year, the matter was not pursued further. Between 1964 and 1975, she was chronically depressed, had frequent anxiety attacks, and was maintained on tranquilizers. She was diagnosed as a "borderline personality with mild retardation." At fifty-seven years of age she was relatively stable but found little in her life to alleviate her feelings of loss and insecurity.

Carla's responses to the TAT were consistent with her feelings of helplessness and lack of support, which she discussed openly with Gutmann. "The stories feature authoritative but rather depriving parents who either refuse help when asked or are absent when their child looks for them. The children are pliable, intropunitive, and conform to parental mandates however arbitrary. There is some evidence of reliance on conversion. Cards which often elicit themes of sadness and hunger instead feature somatic disabilities such as 'The old man is blind.' It is as if the subject avoids dysphoric feelings through the use of somatic denials. She 'blinds' herself to them (as through unconsciousness?)." The circumstances precipitating the conversion symptoms are more like those reported for the Pueblo cases, which also occurred later in life. Clara also differs from the hysterics with fugue states in that she is compliant. Even her TAT contained no themes of rebellion and anger.

The Epileptics

There were twenty-five epileptics with generaliz(d seizures, nine of whom were not interviewed because they were children under seven years of age or alcoholics with seizures consequent on their drinking. There was also one individual whose medical chart was not found. Three of the fifteen cases we interviewed (Carl, Susan, and Mary) are described in the preceding chapter because their hysterical fugue states overshadowed their generalized epileptic seizures. Three epileptics actually committed sibling incest, and four died between 1964 and 1975.

Wilfred always had a turbulent personality and was the only male in the study to commit incest. The second of eight children, he was hit on the head by a rock when he was five. He is said to have lost consciousness at that time and to have behaved abnormally ever since. A paternal cousin has complex partial seizures diagnosed as temporal lobe epilepsy, and his father was a heavy drinker. The father was much older than the mother and was unable to handle Wilfred's temper tantrums, which became more violent as the boy grew. His mother and siblings both pitied and feared him and always let him have his own way. The family converted to Mormonism and Wilfred was sent off to boarding school, where he had poor grades and "hit girls who would not sleep with him."

His first seizure occurred when he was seventeen years old, while he and his sister were herding the sheep. When he did not return home that night, the family searched and found him only a short distance from home, lying on the ground groaning. A lamp was set near him which he proceeded to smash with his fists. After this initial episode, he had one seizure a month, each precipitated by some emotional frustration and heralded by a few hours of variously located headaches. He would fall to the ground, thrash about, then jump to his feet, destroy property, and struggle with anyone close to him. After a seizure he had no memory for anything that had happened and was usually left with a splitting headache.

Two years after the lantern incident, he ran amok for three days. He thrashed about on the ground, scrambled about on all

fours, and howled like a wolf. He grabbed and hit at the people
about him and was finally brought struggling to the hospital,
where he was sedated and flown to a mental hospital for evaluation. There, for the next two days, he was uncommunicative,
thrashed about in bed, and howled. Then, for a week, he behaved normally before having another seizure which was described by the nurses as consisting of contractions of both arm
and leg muscles with facial grimacing, barking sounds, and
snapping of the jaws. Within the hour, he complained of headache and was amnesic for the episode.

The physical exam and an EEG given later were normal. The
psychological report, however, noted a breakdown in associa-
tions, perceptual disorders, blocking, and perseveration (repetition of words or actions). There were also hypochondriacal
ruminations. The diagnostic impression was schizophrenic reaction, and he was sent home "somewhat improved."

He continued to have seizures, which seemed to get worse a
year later when his father died. At this juncture he ran amok
once again and was brought to the hospital for a second time.
"The present admission to this hospital was precipitated by an
outburst of violent behavior during which the patient smashed
up the interior of the hogan, broke down the door, ran away
into the brush, and had to be looked for by the police. Then, in
the emergency room he suddenly leaped from his chair, began
thrashing about on the floor, and again had to be restrained.
The patient himself is amnesic for these events." Once more,
he was flown to a mental hospital where the electroencephalographic examination with Negamide potentiation was still
negative. He was sent home with the plan to enroll him in an
occupational training program.

A year later, at age twenty-two, he was turned over to the
police by the family for repeatedly raping his sister. When his
mother upbraided him for the incestuous act, he became violent, first toward members of the family, then toward himself.
His mother was unable to keep him away from his sister because she was afraid to resist his violent outbursts. Whenever
one of his brothers heard him going toward his sister at night,
he would yell out and Wilfred would quickly leave the hogan.

He made a series of attempts, some successful, on his sister and, whenever thwarted, would become violent. The family finally reported him to the police after he had run off and was later found, his face covered with blood, hitting himself with a hammer.

After his arrest, Wilfred wrote several letters from jail insisting that he would kill himself if he were not allowed to have his sister and that he would never give up his efforts to be with her. The letters that were shown to us were written in a regular, angular, cramped hand that slanted to the left despite the fact that he was right-handed. Stereotypic phrases kept appearing in the letters. Several began, "Hello, I am writing a letter to tell you hello today." The phrase "I mean what I say for God's sake" also appeared several times, oddly glorified with quotation marks. One of the letters described his feelings for his sister: "OK be that way to me, you all don't love me any more. Sis hates me I can see that now. All I do is live in loneliness, misery and lost. How come I can't see Sis anymore? Treat me like a dog. Because of what I have done doesn't mean I can't see Sis anymore does it? That's all I want only Sis, that's all that matters to me. I am not only saying it 'I mean it.' Sis, Sis, only Sis, 'For God's sake.' Maybe you need an interpreter, maybe, maybe not."

Wilfred was sent to a mental hospital, where he remained for several months. For the next eleven years he took antiepileptic medication regularly and was seizure free. He was seen regularly by the hospital mental health staff for a series of psychosomatic complaints and was treated with a variety of tranquilizing drugs for his "personality disorder."

Two years after his return from the mental hospital, Wilfred left home to seek work in Tuba City, but his insomnia, headaches, and pain in the legs and hips soon led him to seek welfare support. In 1975 he was 34 years old and was living in his home community with his Paiute wife. The couple was socially isolated and could count as a friend only a Ute Indian who lived near them. Although Wilfred's wife received Aid to Families of Dependent Children, he was denied welfare.

This case presents several diagnostic problems. It is probable that some of Wilfred's seizures were epileptic despite the fact that two EEGs were within normal limits, because they seem to have been controlled by antiepileptic medications, there is a history of head trauma with loss of consciousness, a cousin has epilepsy, and he loses consciousness during a seizure. Whether these are generalized seizures that have been elaborated by hysterical behaviors or are complex partial epileptic seizures is a moot question. The coexistence of a serious personality problem may have given rise to the purposeful violence and early temper tantrums, obviating the need to postulate the presence of hysteria. The personality problem and the seizures preceded the act of incest. The wolflike behavior, however, although consonant with Navajo beliefs about witchcraft and thus suggestive of a psychic origin, has been observed among epileptics.

The influence of cultural belief should not be overlooked. Navajos believe that witches may assume forms of coyotes, dogs, or other animals while they perform their evil. They are also thought to take control of people who cannot afford ceremonial protection. While a group of witches performs an "evil sing," the individuals in their power are transformed into coyotes and are sent into the countryside to do the witches' bidding.

The case of a middle-aged man brought to the Tuba City hospital illustrates the influence such beliefs can have on pathological behavior. The man in question was poor and became convinced that he was being witched. When more affluent relatives were unwilling to pay for a ceremony, he began to attend peyote meetings in the community. During one of these, he crawled about howling on all fours. Although it was winter and the ground was covered with snow, he ran outside and disappeared into the night. He then terrified the neighborhood by trying to enter various hogans through the smoke hole, all the while howling and walking on all fours. By the time the police brought him to the hospital, his extremities were frostbitten and there was a rope burn about his neck. The police, it seems, shared the belief that he was a wereanimal and refused to lay hands on him. After he was referred to a mental institution, his bizarre behavior disappeared because, he believed, the witches could not harm him as long as he was at some distance from Navajo country. He was diagnosed as schizophrenic and released in a much improved condition. Years later we found him living in an off-reservation bordertown. He had converted to Christianity in the belief that doing so was the only effective protection against the witchcraft, and he was living at a mission where he worked as janitor. Although not actively psychotic, he displayed a flatness of affect and muted motor behavior.

Annie was twenty-six years old in 1964, although we had known her for several years prior to this time. According to her father, her seizures started in 1940, when she was only two years old. She was not brought to medical attention until she was twenty-one, however, at which time she was admitted to the hospital in a semiconscious state and could not respond to questioning. She was sent to an off-reservation hospital for further evaluation, where the neurological and physical exams were unremarkable as was the first EEG. After Metrazol potentiation, however, a second EEG produced spiking at 300 mg which was indicative of a lowered convulsive threshold compatible with idiopathic epilepsy. Annie described her seizures as fainting spells, remembered little about them, and was a poor historian. On occasion, she had episodes of dysuria.

By age seventeen she had a police record. At eighteen she was apprehended while having intercourse with an older, married brother who had a long history of drinking but no evidence of a convulsive disorder. The succeeding years were marked by a series of arrests for drunken and disorderly conduct with many references to promiscuousness. Two episodes took place during the 1960s that were of such tragic and gargantuan proportions as to warrant description here.

The first was told us by the manager of a trading post adjacent to the reservation where liquor was sold. It appears that Annie became intoxicated and began selling her favors to anyone who would pay her with a pint of wine. Soon the trader saw a line of men forming behind the corral. His interest quickened; he started to keep count as men kept arriving throughout the afternoon and early evening. He believed that she must have passed out after a while because the men no longer bothered to leave a bottle of wine as payment. The trader was able

to count over sixty customers and believed that, as he did not
start counting until after he noticed a line had formed and was
unable to keep counting after it got dark, there would easily
have been as many as a hundred men involved.

The second incident came directly to our notice after Annie
was found one morning in the plaza of a Hopi village. It appears
that a group of Hopi men got her drunk and gang-raped her.
Then, in the early morning hours, they left her against the wall
of a house on the village plaza with her dress thrown back over
her head and an ear of blue corn protruding from her vagina.
There she was found by the women of the village when they
came to draw water from the public tap. She was immediately
called "Blue Corn Girl," and became the object of much joking
despite the fact that some of the men were married and their
identities known to all.

In 1963, when she was twenty-five years old, Annie left the
reservation to live with an Anglo in a bordertown. She told us
that she was happy for the first time in her life. Nevertheless,
the couple drank heavily and soon separated. Over the next
three years she took her antiepileptic medication erratically
and suffered frequent seizures, especially when in jail. Between
1964 and 1970, she drank heavily and had bouts of aggressive
and psychotic behavior. In 1967, she was hospitalized because
of a severe psychotic reaction caused by her drinking. No diagnosis of schizophrenia was made at that time, however. Her
father died in 1967 and, a year later when she was thirty years
old, she gave birth to an illegitimate child and was fitted with
an intrauterine device. The next year she contracted active tuberculosis and was sent to a sanitorium but was returned home
because of her aggressive outbursts. After this return, she refused all medications and, two months later, was found frozen
to death in a nearby border town. Her drinking, it seemed to us,
was an act of desperation and her death self-willed.

Annie's father claimed that he had always been too poor to
pay for the ceremonial treatments his daughter needed. By his
account, a hand trembler told them that Annie's mother had
gathered some corn pollen and broken a prenatal tabu and that
this was the cause of the seizures. While still a very young
child, the family had a short ritual performed for her which

included two small sand paintings of male and female corn bee-
tles. After this, however, no further efforts were made and, it
will be recalled, Annie was not even brought to medical attention until she was twenty-one years old.

The community believed, of course, that Annie was *'iich'ah*,
but not because of the mother's act or because of the sibling
incest which took place many years later. Instead, it was said
that her seizures were caused by her father who had transgressed a tabu before Annie's birth. Although we were never
able to learn exactly what the father had done, it appears to
have been serious because he was forced to leave his home
community the year that Annie's seizures began. There was
reason for the family to guard its reputation closely; it was one
of a group of related families with a tradition of marrying back
into father's clan. In addition, theirs was the only kin group in
the area with a *nádleeh* (transvestite). The family was not well
off despite the fact that Annie's paternal grandfather was a singer, that two of his sons followed in his footsteps, and another
became a politician.

Betty's seizures began soon after the death of her daughter,
when she was twenty-one years old. After that, they occurred
monthly, usually in the evening. Her sister believed there was
some relationship with the menses. The spells began with a
feeling of pressure on the back of the head, after which she
would fall to the ground with symmetrical trembling movements. Her eyes would stare or turn to one side. She would be
incontinent, turn blue about the mouth, and clamp her jaw
shut tightly. These episodes lasted anywhere from a few minutes to a few hours. Occasionally she would get up after a seizure, sing songs, and hallucinate that someone was coming
after her. She had also experienced weekly bouts of psychotic
behavior during which she became paranoid and violent. We
felt the seizures were probably epileptic combined with some
complex hysterical fugue states. When we interviewed her in
1964, she was thirty years old, had a history of drinking and
promiscuity, and was the mother of four illegitimate children.
She was still incontinent of urine, as were her sixteen-year-old
daughter and seven-year-old son.

Her family claim that, while drunk, Betty committed incest with a clan "brother" and, on another occasion, had intercourse with a man who had not purified himself after hunting. Her maternal grandfather, who was a retired stargazer and hand trembler, said that the *bé'ékǫ́ǫ́zz* ritual should be performed for the incest and a full Mountainway for the contact with the hunter. Neither of these had been performed because, according to her parents, she did not have a husband to help pay for the ceremonies. Her family, in their own words, were just "putting up with her."

Late in 1964, Betty was admitted to hospital for her drinking. She complained of right upper quadrant pains and was found to have a fatty liver. Cirrhosis was suspected, but she never returned for the tests that had been scheduled. A year later, she was admitted complaining of intermittent fever for one month and, again, she failed to return for the scheduled work-up. Then, only two weeks later, at age forty-two, she was found dead at her parents home after a bout of drinking. No autopsy was performed, and no cause of death was entered into her record.

As in Annie's case, there are a number of unanswered questions. That Betty was seen in Tuba City hospital for epilepsy is certain because we found the diagnostic sheet in the central office in Window Rock. There was, however, no reference to seizures in her medical chart, although her parents maintained that she was brought to hospital because of them; thus, we were unable to verify when they first appeared. It seemed unlikely that the epileptic seizures started only at age twenty-one after the death of a daughter. It is more likely they preceded the drinking and the incest by some years and that it was the hysterical seizures which began after the death of her daughter. By denying an early onset, the family could attribute the epilepsy to the known incest and thus avoid suspicion that they were to blame.

Robert. Betty and Annie were from families of ceremonialists, neither had any signs performed for them, and both died. A similar pattern may be discerned in the case of Robert, whose father was a singer and whose mother was an herbalist. He was diagnosed as epileptic when he was eleven, six years after he had contracted tuberculosis meningitis. The seizures were observed by physicians, and the EEG and neurological exam were abnormal. His seizures were frequent, lasted up to fifteen minutes, and involved fecal incontinence, tetany, and cyanosis. They were, fortunately, well controlled by antiepileptic medication, and he was able to live at home.

Robert's parents preferred to keep him out of school and to care for him at home, although this care did not involve ceremonial treatments. They refused to give their consent for him to be sent to a special school away from the reservation when he was sixteen years old. He rebelled by taking his medications erratically, with the inevitable reoccurrence of seizures. After four months, he attempted suicide by taking an overdose of his medications, which resulted in loss of consciousness. For a year and a half he had numerous seizures and temper tantrums. He ran away from home three times and, on the last occasion, he was found in an off-reservation city in a disoriented state. Finally pursuaded, his parents allowed to him to leave for school where, four months after his arrival, he was found dead after falling from a window. The records and correspondence did little to elucidate the circumstances but, in light of the suicide attempt, we believe death by suicide is very likely.

Laura, the fourth to die, was a 31-year-old, obese, and mentally sluggish woman, who had epileptic seizures and some bouts of bizarre behavior thought to have been caused by organic brain syndrome. Although brought to medical attention at age fifteen, she was said to have had seizures since infancy. No seizure had been seen by a physician, and there was no EEG report in her chart. She had been seen in a referral hospital, however, and had also been in a mental institution. Physicians had observed postictal states involving stuporousness and, at times, bizarre behavior. The general impression at that time was of chronic brain syndrome with mild mental deficiency. A psychological etiology was ruled out because she responded well to antiepileptic medication.

Descriptions of the seizures were obtained from the family. There was no aura. The prodrome consisted of jerking motions of the lips and legs. She complained of headache and a generally "funny" feeling before falling and losing consciousness for about eight minutes. Foaming at the mouth was also said to occur. Postictally she slept for some time or was stuporous. Except when taking medication, she was never free of seizures for more than one month.

Episodes of "strange" behavior were also noted by family, police, and hospital personnel, which may have been hysterical or due to the organic brain syndrome. An account of one such episode is typical. Once, when she was 25 years old, she became agitated, began cursing, and became violent toward a visiting welfare worker. The police were called for, and she was put into jail. According to the arresting officer, she was confused as to location. Although somnolent that night, she became more active the next day and began singing. This activity was continued, more or less constantly, for five days. Once, when in the café where the prisoners were taken to eat, she stripped to the waist to attract the attention of the male prisoners, became somewhat violent, and had to be restrained.

Laura's mother is said to have died from *yistezh*, a sexual infection of the genitals caused by Rabid Coyote. A hand trembler diagnosed a Coyote etiology for Laura when she was still a baby, but the appropriate rituals had never been performed. Instead she was treated with Shootingway, Windway, and Lifeway.

Laura appeared to be doing reasonably well until, three months after our interview, she was found dead about a mile from her home. No autopsy was performed, no cause of death was noted in the chart, and the family maintained they did not know how she died. We think it possible that her death was due to the disease itself although, admittedly, we do not have much information on which to base this opinion.

Anna was orphaned when a young child and experienced seizures since infancy. There was no history of seizures among other family members. She was separated from her siblings, who were adopted by a maternal aunt and who developed normally, married, and had children of their own. The relatives who took Anna into their home treated her poorly, and it was not until she was a young adult that a kinsman who was a prominent politician arranged for her to live with a blind, old clan "grandfather." It was only after this living arrangement had been made that Anna was brought to medical attention and was able to have Navajo sings performed. This was in 1945, when she was nineteen years of age. At this time she was diagnosed as having epilepsy. Some of her seizures were observed by physicians, who called them conversion reactions.

Her seizures occur twice each month and consist of fear and extreme palpitation. She lies face down and her "grandfather" hears a grunting cry. Apparently she loses consciousness and thrashes around before getting up in a twilight state. Often she recovers to find herself walking about outside the hogan. There is no incontinence or tongue biting, but she has wrenched earrings from her ear leaving a still visible hiatus. The twilight states may last two hours. Only the blind "grandfather" has been present during these seizures. Levy and a physician observed one seizure which was clearly hysterical. Unfortunately, the description was not entered into the chart. As Levy recalled it, she was trembling all over with her head turned to one side. She was referred to another hospital for evaluation, where she was seizure-free and the EEG and neurological exam were negative. In light of at least a twenty-year history of regularly occurring spells, we doubt these seizures are purely hysterical.

She had been kept in a virtual state of slavery by her relatives, made to do all the hard work, and, according to some older people in the community, forced to prostitute herself. There were several notes in her medical chart mentioning that she was assaulted and had contracted gonorrhea. Many in the community believe that she lived in an incestuous relationship with her clan grandfather and that this was the cause of her seizures. Anna and her "grandfather" believe that her father had practiced gambling witchcraft, which ultimately caused the death of both parents as well as the seizures. Because her father used a sand painting to work his witchcraft, several sand paintings from as many sings have been made for her. She has also had several Windways, a Shootingway, and an Evilway.

After interviewing her and administering a Thematic Apperception Test in 1964 when she was forty-two years old, Gutmann noted her "mistrustful, anaclitic-paranoid attitude." The hogan itself betrayed Anna's compulsive habits. Everything was spic and span. Hospital appointments and menses were meticulously recorded on a wall calendar. There were lists of food staples with their prices carefully marked. Some peculiar photocollages of volcanoes and panthers cut from *Life* magazine served as decoration. The TAT was "very much of a conversion protocol. She spoke of physical states such as headaches when referring to cards where others experience affects. A rather isolated and isolating person. There were breakthroughs of intense death concerns; the old man will come apart 'like an overripe melon,' or 'owls will eat a dead man.' Impression: A schizoid person with paranoid and compulsive trends. Essentially she has little or no trust in others; that they will stay around, be helpful, or that they won't 'fall apart.'" She withdraws from any traffic with the wider world into her hogan where, through compulsive neatness and bizarre packrat forms of ordering, she maintains the illusion of being in control of and central to her relevant universe."

Anna continued to experience seizures between 1964 and 1975. She was also seen regularly by the mental health staff. Once she complained of being raped by a man she was able to identify but, although she was bruised, there was no way to verify the statement and she did not lodge a formal complaint. She tends to feel depressed, to feel aches all over her body, and to be fatigued much of the time.

All of these cases came from the Tuba City area. This does not mean that Fort Defiance is free of these problems but that our data from there are less detailed because we were unable to recontact the patients or follow them over the years as we were able to do in Tuba City. We did find one young woman from the Fort Defiance Service Unit who had committed incest, but we were unable to find out whether it was a case of sibling incest or when it happened.

Sibling Incest

The three cases of incest represent 27 percent of all epileptics found in the Tuba City Service Unit and a third of those with generalized seizures. This proportion seemed unusually high, and we were led to conduct a field survey in one of the communities to determine the number of epileptics not identified by our case-finding methods. Informants were able to identify three additional cases with little trouble (Table 8.1).

Case 4 is the case of incest already described that took place around the turn of the century. The woman experienced a single episode of fainting. The brother was asymptomatic. He left the community and, ultimately, married a Paiute woman. Case 5 involved an epileptic girl who was seduced by a clan sibling. Despite the fact that she had suffered from seizures since childhood, no seizure-specific diagnosis was made until after the act of incest. The *bé'ékáz̨* ritual was performed, although the family believes her disease cannot be cured unless the Mothway is performed. The man left the area soon after the relationship was discovered. Case 6 involved clan siblings who committed incest by mutual consent. The couple lived together in the home community and, in 1964, had exhibited no untoward symptoms for nine years. We were unable to contact this couple and so know nothing about the closeness of the clan relationship, their relatives, or the history and description of an episode of "acute brain syndrome with confused state" found in the male partner's medical chart.

From these few cases it is difficult to generalize. One pattern that emerges clearly, however, is that one member of each pair

Table 8.1. Sibling and Clan Incest in the Tuba City Service Unit

Cases	Sex	Diagnosis	Incest	Partner's Symptoms
		STUDY GROUP		
1. Annie	F	Epilepsy	Sibling	None
2. Wilfred	M	Epilepsy	Sibling	None
3. Betty	F	Epilepsy	Clan	None
		COMMUNITY SURVEY		
4.	F	Hysteria?	Sibling	None
5.	F	Epilepsy	Clan	None
6.	M	Brain Syndrome	Clan	None

is always asymptomatic. We suspect also that the existence of childhood epilepsy among females creates a self-fulfilling prophecy. An epileptic woman has no social value so that, unless isolated and protected by her family, she is exposed to rape and sexual exploitation even by close relatives. This happened to three epileptic women, and even in Wilfred's case the epilepsy preceded the incest.

Even more than others, the families of ceremonialists appear to be traumatized by the presence of an epileptic child and tend not to seek treatment for him or her. We think this is because they have more to lose by having the condition become known in the community. Three of the four deaths and two of the three cases of incest in the study population were children from ceremonialists' families.

The hysterics in our group, as predicted, did not reproduce the signs of the epileptic major motor seizure. The case of the elderly informant identified in the community survey is interesting because it is the only case in which incest preceded the seizures. Taken together, the cases support the view of the singer who told us that seizures cause incest as often as incest produces seizures—and both represent the effects of Coyote contamination.

CHAPTER 9

Ambivalence, Anxiety,

and Incest

Moth madness is still the apical Navajo disease, although why the incest it signifies is the focus of such anxiety and concern remains to be explained. Before addressing this question, let us review our speculative reconstruction of the development of the incest prohibition. When the Apacheans arrived in the Southwest, they had in all likelihood a general proscription against familial incest that included marriage to close blood relatives. The tabu was expressed by the myth, ubiquitous among western tribes, of Coyote's seduction of his daughter, and incest was equated with witchcraft (Schmerla 1931). If, as many anthropologists believe, matrilineal descent developed subsequent to the adoption of agriculture and contact with the matrilineal western Pueblos, there would have been no compelling reason to create a new prohibition against sibling incest—although there may have been reason to extend the preexisting tabu to include a prohibition against clan endogamy. The matrilineal Western Apaches, we recall, have done just this. Familial incest and all irregular sex with members of the opposite sex were linked by these groups with incest and looked upon with horror. Incest with close blood relatives was thought to be worse than that between clan relatives, and the most repugnant of all was father-daughter and sibling incest. Among the Navajos, however, sibling and clan incest have been given a position of great importance. Father-daughter incest, on the other hand, is prominent neither in myth nor as a cause of disease. Moreover, the myths of Mothway and Frenzy-witchcraftway are of Pueblo origin. We recall also that the Pueblos do not have well-defined prohibitions against incest. The Hopis can hardly conceive of someone committing incest and do not have very clear ideas about what the consequences would be. The Zunis have no specific punishment for sibling incest but believe that clan incest will cause a natural catastrophe. In sum, the Navajos borrowed myths and symbols from the Pueblos but not their beliefs about incest and its consequences.

We have speculated that these borrowings took place during the period of intense Puebloization which lasted from 1690 to about 1770. The myth details the untoward consequences of not accepting marriage offers from the various foreign groups with whom the Butterfly people came into contact on their wanderings. Moth madness was the punishment for community endogamy which included marriage into father's, shared fathers', and, possibly, the grandparents' clans.[1] This proscription was developed to promote the integration of the various groups of Pueblo refugees in the fairly large permanent settlements which formed at that time. But, as the need to integrate numerous descent groups within the larger polity lessened during the nineteenth century, the prohibition was narrowed to include only sibling incest and marriage to classificatory siblings— that is, matrilateral parallel cousins who are members of the same clan and who are called siblings.

The troubled lives of Navajo epileptics and the number of them who do commit incest suggest that the sanction is more than an historical remnant, that, in fact, it remains charged with emotion. But what evidence is there to suggest that familial incest is of special concern and, if it is, why is father-daughter incest not given an equally important position in Navajo myth and disease theory?

Incest and Sexual Ambivalence

We think the shift to pastoralism had three consequences that fostered anxiety and a fear of incest. The dispersal of the population and the adoption of a seminomadic lifestyle increased the isolation of families, thereby weakening many social controls. Opportunity and weak social controls, however, although preconditions for incest, were not in our opinion sufficient reason for such a severe punishment to retain its force for almost two centuries. This was effected by the third consequence of the shift to pastoralism—a gender conflict that developed as the society shifted from one in which the position of women was secure to one in which males managed the economy and contended with women for their prerogatives. This conflict exacerbated an ambivalent attitude toward women developed during early childhood, so that frustrated adult males turned their attention to less threatening younger females.

Overcrowding, proximity, the absence of suitable sex partners outside the family, and frustrated marital relations have all been identified as factors predisposing to incest and were certainly characteristic of Navajo life until very recent times (Masters 1963:79–84). On the other hand, although many North American tribes lived in scattered encampments that were isolated for much of the year, recorded accounts do not suggest that incest was a source of much anxiety. Some tribes knew only sibling incest, others only that between father and daughter. There were tribes with knowledge of both kinds and groups like the Pueblos who could hardly conceive of it happening. Similar variability is found in the beliefs about the causes of incest and the sanctions against it. The north Alaskan Eskimos, for example, had never heard of an incestuous relationship between brother and sister and only one instance of father-daughter incest could be recalled, although that was between a man and his daughter by adoption. "When the wife died, the daughter remained with her adoptive father as his wife. People said of this man, 'He should be ashamed' and of the girl that 'she had no pride.' While no group action would be taken in such a case, the guilty parties could be made to feel the full force of adverse public opinion. When the girl's adoptive father died, she was claimed by another family in marriage. It is thus clear that there was no lasting stigma in such cases" (R.F. Spencer 1959:76).

The Cheyenne had a political system that included lesser and greater chiefs, as well as warrior societies with police functions. Yet Llewellyn and Hoebel (1941:178–81) concluded that incest was a family matter and there was no direct public legal sanction against it, although ostracism often forced offenders to leave the band. Similarly, the Comanches did not rationalize the tabu and the only social controls were ridicule and ostracism (Hoebel 1940:108–10).

The Kaska Indians, Athabascan speakers of western Canada, believed that witchcraft and incest caused insanity. "Overwhelmed by shame and guilt, an unhappy man might tear off his penis or leap into the fire. Most grievous of all was incest between brother and sister" (Honigman 1954:90–91). The single case reported resulted in the murder of the offending brother by his sister's husband. This, however, was a double offense, both incest and adultery, itself a special concern of the Kaska. "In the presence of an economy that forced men to leave their wives in camp while they hunted, plenty of opportunity for adultery existed. Chronic jealousy and suspicion haunted husbands" (Honigman 1954:91). The Apaches permitted the killing of one or both offenders by relatives. They also accused mature males of witchcraft and, as long as the witch was not greatly feared, executed him (Opler 1965:59, 250; Goodwin 1969:416–24, 427).[2]

The question is whether the strength of the sanction and the perceived seriousness of the crime are functions of the degree of family isolation. The answer, unfortunately, is not forthcoming from the data, which are lacking for many tribes and too briefly reported for others, so that intertribal comparisons cannot be made in anything but an impressionistic manner. The most commonly reported sanction is community disapproval, often resulting in the offender leaving the group. In the event that both parties persisted in the union and established a new household, however, the community was powerless to act.

Some questions are unanswerable given the paucity of the data. Does a concern with sibling incest indicate that father-daughter incest is less frequent? Are matrilineal societies more likely to be concerned about sibling than father-daughter incest? Is the severity of the punishment a gauge of the crime's prevalence or even of the level of concern?

The prevalence of various forms of incest is impossible to determine. Communities can only know the cases that become public when the partners "marry" and form a new family, or when one of the offenders is forced and charges the other with the crime, or when a third party discovers the offense and announces it publicly. Almost all Indian accounts cast the male in the role of perpetrator, yet incest initiated by the female is the least likely form to come to public attention. Still, there are cases of sibling incest which seem to have been desired by both partners, and there is no reason to believe that there were no instances of women who seduced their brothers or their sons. With these caveats in mind, let us turn to the evidence supporting the argument that, among the Navajos, family isolation, weak social controls, and the shifting sexual division of labor fostered ambivalent feelings toward the opposite sex that suffused the incestuous impulse, making it more anxiety-provoking than it was among tribes whose way of life had been stable for longer periods of time.

Clyde Kluckhohn believed that tensions generated between members of the extended family were "hypertrophied by the emotional inbreeding which the geographic isolation of Navaho households makes almost inevitable" (Kluckhohn 1962:93). When the margin of subsistence is slim, cooperation is an imperative. Witchcraft serves to release hostilities generated within the group by displacing and projecting aggression onto persons outside the immediate kin group.

The members of a consumption group unavoidably see a very great deal of each other, and this intercourse is not restricted to the necessities of economic co-operation. But the nearest other consumption group will usually be at least a mile away and is likely to be several miles to ten miles away. This means, especially during the winter months and during periods of intense economic activity, that contact with outsiders is limited; chances to "let off steam" about grudges, suspicions, jealousies to persons who are not emotionally involved are infrequent. . . . The result is a strong tendency toward involvement in a morbid nexus of emotional sensitivities from which there is little escape through socially approved patterns. (Kluckhohn 1962:93).

Kluckhohn used the term "consumption group" to refer to the coresident extended family, or camp. Camps were comprised of anywhere from one to six or eight households. A "typical," multihousehold camp included a parent couple and their unmarried children, one or more married daughters and their husbands and children, and occasional dependents (the elderly or incapacitated). In the 1930s, a survey of 3,700 camps—almost the entire Navajo population—showed that 53 percent consisted of independent (not extended) families, over 80 percent of which were nuclear—that is, composed of a married couple and their dependent children (Aberle 1961:187). Thus, isolated family groups were small nuclear families as often as not.

Although Kluckhohn was primarily concerned with analyzing the functions of witchcraft, he recognized that social isolation fosters intense attachments as well as conflict and hostility. He wondered why it was always a sibling who was mentioned in Navajo accounts as the relative killed by the witch initiate (Kluckhohn 1962:102–4). When informants told of wereanimals, they often mentioned that the witch was recognized as a real or clan sister. Kluckhohn also recognized that the unconscious feelings were ambivalent and noted that, when incest was mentioned, it almost always involved siblings. Strong ambivalent feelings are likely to generate more anxiety than direct feelings of attraction, although both would have to be repressed. Much of the hostility, he believed, could be accounted for by early socialization practices:

The Navajo baby receives a maximum of gratification. The mother gives the baby her breast whenever it cries, day or night. The baby is assured of the constant physical nearness of the mother and receives a great deal of actual fondling. But when a new sibling is born all of this changes—and usually rather abruptly. It is hardly surprising that hostile impulses should be generated against the displacing rival. . . . There are, of course, also many factors which promote positive feeling toward siblings. The unusual strength of the prohibitions on physical contact between siblings of opposite sex suggests strong need for controlling libidinous impulses between brother and sister. (Kluckhohn 1962:103)

Among the Pueblos social controls were of two types. The Hopis relied almost exclusively on gossip and community disapproval; the priestly societies of the other Pueblos had the authority to execute witches and to expel deviants from the village. None of the conditions thought to foster incest were present in the densely populated and tightly controlled Pueblo communities. By contrast, although Navajo myths contain many references to chiefs, head chiefs, and chiefs' councils, political organization during the late nineteenth century was minimal. By the time anthropologists began to investigate this area of Navajo life, the aboriginal system had disappeared and accounts given by aged informants were confused and contradictory, often mixing mythological with ethnographic elements. During the years immediately prior to the establishment of the reservation, there appear to have been leaders of vaguely defined communities who had no coercive power but whose recognized leadership qualities gave them powers of persuasion (K. Spencer, 1947:76–81). Gossip was an inadequate form of social control in a scattered population. What remained was the fear of being thought a witch and the threat of supernaturally caused disease, and these had to be of a fearful nature if they were to be effective against the strong ambivalent feelings generated within the family group.

The cases of incest we have presented show the use of a variety of social control mechanisms.[3] Two incest offenders were reported to the police, indicating some degree of reliance on modern forms of external control. At the other extreme, an incestuous couple who established a new family were left alone, the community being unwilling to proceed against them formally. We cannot know how many potential instances of incest were deterred by fear of the consequences. That one woman was so anxiety-ridden as to have a fainting spell that brought the matter to her family's attention suggests that the sanctions were powerful. Parents of epileptic children often tried to keep the condition secret and refused to provide ceremonial treatment for them because they feared the community would accuse the parents of incest or the father of witchcraft. Those few epileptics who had committed incest were dramatic examples of the consequences in store for potential offenders.

Incestuous urges may become particularly anxiety provoking if attitudes toward the opposite sex are ambivalent—that is, if the attraction is mixed with hostility and fear. Excessive attraction may be repressed and masked by feelings of hostility which permit a person to distance himself from the object of his desire. If, however, hostility is already present, there is the danger of producing excessive aggression within the family. The development of ambivalent feelings toward the mother and siblings has already been discussed. Initially the child is indulged, given the breast on demand, held and fondled. Dependence and attraction develop during the earliest years, but the suddenness and completeness of the displacement when the next child arrives generates hostility and mistrust. Older sisters are often assigned the task of caring for the child so displaced. As the older sibling already harbors resentment of her own displacement, her behavior toward her charge alternates between affection and hostility, thus prolonging and intensifying the ambivalent emotions. Opportunities for contacts with other children are limited to matrilateral parallel cousins in the same camp who are equated with siblings.[4]

Boyer (1979) has described the stages of child rearing, sibling rivalries, and ambivalent attitudes toward the mother and of the mother toward her children among the Mescalero Apaches. Although he does not mention that incestuous urges are salient among them, in other respects the Mescalero basic personality is almost identical to that of the Navajo presented here. Whether the Apaches also have a heightened concern about incest cannot be answered with the data at hand. There is, however, reason to believe that the Navajos' shift to pastoralism generated sex role conflicts that exacerbated the ambivalent attitudes toward parents and siblings created by child-rearing practices.

The Navajos are unique among North American Indian societies in having been pastoralists. Pastoralism is a male-managed subsistence pursuit associated with patrilocal or virilocal residence and patrilineal descent the world over (Textor 1967:printout #61). Moreover, according to Lowie (1961:193), the status of women in these societies is "almost uniformly one of decided and absolute inferiority." The Navajos' shift from agriculture to pastoralism, which began only during the late eighteenth century and which coincided with an increase in raiding and warfare, elevated the managerial roles of men in a society that was already matrilineal and in which women enjoyed considerable control over the use and distribution of resources.

The position of males was made difficult by the fact that, after marriage, they took up residence with their wives' families. The young, married male was in many respects a servant in his wife's camp. He took orders from his father-in-law who directed herding operations, while the women dominated the domestic sphere. His kinsmen lived too far away to provide emotional support or to take his part in marital quarrels. The authority of his mother-in-law could not be questioned, and opportunities for argument were curtailed by the practice of mother-in-law avoidance. While this maintained distance between potential adversaries and lessened the open expression of hostility, it also made the husband, who was not allowed to be present in the same dwelling as his mother-in-law, a stranger in his own home. Men very often found relaxation only when they were away on trading or hunting expeditions or attending ceremonials.

The position of the woman in her own family was more secure. The relationship of children and fathers was warm, the affection less warm than that for mothers, perhaps, but also containing less suppressed resentment (Leighton and Kluckhohn 1947:98). For women, who remained at home after marriage, fathers were often present and supportive, although there was the feeling that they were less dependable because of their many absences. Still, until recently, marriages were arranged by the parents and girls were not infrequently forced to marry older men who held little attraction for them. Whatever the women's feelings and attitudes toward men, and they must have been ambivalent, they were most easily handled by withdrawing into the protective circle of mother, aunts, and sisters, thus further excluding the husband. Not surprisingly, divorce was frequent, men spent much of their time away, and only those who could persevere for ten to twenty years could hope to assume a position of authority in their wives' families.

Evidence of sexual difficulties and hostility is found in myths, early Navajo autobiographies, and the patterns of suicide and homicide. We have already noted that the story of the separation of the sexes occupies a pivotal position in the Navajo creation myth. It is accounted for in one of two ways: either the women come to believe they have no further need for men, or the men are angered after the women are unfaithful to them. In both versions the male is rejected. In the discussion of the impending separation, the men argue that they do most of the productive work. They clear the fields, help the women till them, plant the crops, hunt, and help and guide the women in all their labors. The women reply that they do more work tilling fields, gathering seeds and fruits, making clothing, caring for children, and cooking.[5] Son of Old Man Hat (1967:48–49), born in 1868, finally comes to realize in old age that the economically productive work performed by men is more than equaled by the suffering of women who bear babies, raise many children, and care for the man who "only makes a woman suffer."

In the creation myth, the relationship between husband and wife is revealed in the many accounts of quarrels arising from infidelity (K. Spencer 1947:35–39). Ethnographic accounts also refer to the ubiquitousness of infidelity and marital discord (Leighton and Kluckhohn 1947:83–86). During the separation, men and women masturbate with a variety of objects, and Coyote secretly crosses over to the women and, in a frenzy of lustfulness, practices cunnilingus and copulates indiscriminately with his sisters. The message is that uncontrolled lust is socially disruptive. Many beliefs and practices indicate fear and distrust of sex. For example, Navajos do not expose their genitals to the view of members of either sex because it is widely believed that whoever looks at a woman's vagina will be struck by lightning and that viewing the glans penis will cause sickness.

While still a boy, Son of Old Man Hat (1967:47–49) tells his mother that he doesn't want to have anything to do with women who are not already related to him, "because she is not my mother." His mother explains that when he grows up he will have a wife and that when she wants to leave him he will cry and hang on to her just as if she were his mother. "That's the way they think of each other, just like father and mother." She then goes on to explain how, as soon as a man marries, "he may start beating his wife, and they'll begin to have a quarrel every once in a while. . . . It's pretty dangerous to have a wife or a husband. Some men when they have wives, may kill their wives or may get killed by them, and some commit suicide."

Noticeably absent from the Navajos' conceptualization of sex is the idea that sexual indulgence depletes the male's strength and the concomitant value placed on chastity and self-denial. A Navajo would not understand the Cheyenne who proudly told how, after the birth of his first child, he lived fifteen years in perfect harmony with his wife without any sex relations and without strain (Llewellyn and Hoebel 1941:263). Sex and fecundity were desirable; the urge was not to be repressed. Rather, relationships between the sexes were thought to be difficult and fraught with danger at best; unbridled lust, because it precluded the possibility of creating harmonious marital relations, was to be guarded against at all costs.

Marital trouble, especially jealousy, was found to be the most frequent cause of suicide, accounting for 47 percent of all suicides committed on the reservation between 1954 and 1963 (Levy 1965). Thirteen males committed suicide for every female. During the 1940s, 32 percent of suicides were preceded by a murder, and in 78 percent of these the wife was the victim. After 1954, only 7 percent of suicides were associated with murder, but violence of all types was found in 43 percent of the cases, with almost all the violence aimed at the wife.

Alcohol lessens inhibitions, and the question arises whether murder and suicide have increased over the years as the use of intoxicants became commonplace. The consumption of alcohol increased rapidly after 1940; yet the suicide rate seems to have been relatively stable from the early years of the reservation through the 1960s. Moreover, the Navajo rate has, until very recently, always been slightly lower than that of the nation as a whole. Although the association of alcohol with suicide rose from 9 percent in the 1940s to 47 percent between 1954 and 1963, the proportion of suicides preceded by murder decreased precipitously. Not only does suicide reflect the strains in the marital situation, it is also an act of passive aggression. The dominant pattern is for a married, active male between thirty-five and forty years of age to kill himself in or near the dwelling so that his ghost may contaminate his wife and her relatives.

Until recently the Hopi suicide rate and the ratio of male to female offenders were about the same as the Navajos'. The precipitating stresses, however, were quite different. The Hopi suicide was the child of a disapproved marriage (Levy, Kunitz, and Henderson, in press). Hopi villages were endogamous, and marriages were alliances between lineages of roughly equal status. Although the husband lived with his wife's family and worked their fields, his family lived close by, could take his part in family quarrels, and provide him refuge when emotions ran high. Moreover, the husband continued to fulfill his ceremonial obligations in his own village. This balance was upset when marriage brought in a man from another village. Family quarrels were intense as the wife's family took her side against the husband, and there was often considerable pressure exerted to have her terminate the marriage. The men, under these circumstances, could gain no status in their wives' village and often took to drink. The children grew up in a stressful atmosphere and, as they reached adulthood, there were many conflicts between sons and their fathers. Sons committed suicide to shame their fathers, and many became alcoholics. There was also a pattern of family suicide epidemics triggered when a murder was committed by a father or brother. In these cases, the reaction of siblings was one of shame. Thus, although marital stress was an important ingredient, sexual jealousy does not appear to have been one of the major motives despite the fact that infidelity was frequent.

Father-Daughter Incest

To the extent that family isolation and sexual ambivalence increase anxiety and incestuous impulses, we would expect father-daughter incest to be treated in much the same manner as sibling incest. This form of incest, however, is not said to be the cause of a named disease like moth madness, nor does there seem to be any specified supernatural sanction. Nevertheless, we believe that it was a real problem throughout the years when the Navajos were pastoralists. Although none of the epileptics in the study seem to have been seduced by their fathers and we did not ask about this in the community survey, our impression is that the Tuba City police records contain about as many cases of father-daughter as sibling incest.

Among the types of preferred polygynous unions, marriage of a man to a woman and her daughter was common because it provided some inducement for younger men to marry older women who needed their labor. It also legitimatized sexual relations between a mature male and a very young woman who could give him solace when he felt rejected and frustrated by his first wife. Such marriages could, on occasion, function as a permissible substitute for father-daughter incest, perhaps even precluding it. Old Mexican, who was born in 1866, married two stepdaughters who were "given" to him by his first wife to appease him (Dyk 1947). As the younger women were no more faithful than their mother, however, and as Old Mexican himself was not averse to committing adultery, it is not clear just how successful the arrangement was. Men did, however, initiate relations with their stepdaughters without their wives' permission and some committed incest. The case of Hiram, who seduced his stepdaughter, two daughters, and four granddaughters, reveals something about the quality of the relationships and the powerlessness of the community to prevent them.[6]

Hiram was born sometime between 1882 and 1892 and lived all his life in the same community on the western Navajo reservation. When he was about twenty-five years old, he married a widow with children who belonged to a "branch" of his own clan. Although in Hiram's community today they are assigned to separate clan groups, in most areas of the reservation this marriage would be forbidden. Thus, it is possible that their marriage had a taint of incest about it from the very beginning.

Hiram had four children by this marriage, before he seduced and impregnated his oldest stepdaughter who was then between nine and fourteen years of age. When his wife discovered this, she left him in disgust. Hiram and his stepdaughter lived together for over twenty years and had twelve children, eight of whom survived. When the oldest daughter was about fourteen years old, Hiram seduced her several times, threatening to kill her if she told anyone about it. The girl, however, informed her mother who told the police. The daughter was willing to testify and Hiram, now fifty-eight, was sentenced to two years imprisonment in a federal penitentiary. At the trial, Hiram's wife (i.e., his stepdaughter) testified that "he was always talking of killing someone," and she felt "he would kill some of them and himself before this crime was finished."

Three years after his return, he was again charged with incest in tribal court and served a sentence in a reservation jail. After this, his wife left him and remarried. Some years later one of Hiram's daughters, Bernice, was convicted of committing incest with a first cousin, her mother's sister's son.

For the next seven years, Hiram lived much of the time with his daughters, including Bernice and her "husband." Then, when he was in his late seventies, complaints about his behavior were again made to the police. The investigation revealed he had been having sexual relations with Bernice for a number of years, with two of her daughters, and with two other granddaughters between seven and ten years of age. Evidence was gathered from the girls and from a neighbor who had witnessed one of the acts.

The descriptions obtained by the police attest to the hostile and punitive nature of Hiram's sexuality. One granddaughter said that Hiram would chase her on horseback whenever she was alone herding sheep and that he forced her to go out herding so that he could find her alone. Even though she tried to evade him, he would follow her tracks and "hunt her down." He would fondle her so roughly that she would cry. She witnessed Hiram forcibly rape her younger sister despite her cries for help and also saw him force her mother in the hogan many times. Her sister confirmed this testimony. Two other granddaughters claimed that Hiram stayed with them for three months, during which time he would penetrate either with his finger or his penis, hurting them badly. He always threatened to whip or kill them if they told anyone. One neighbor told the police that she had come upon the old man having intercourse with one of the girls. He had her standing on her head with her legs apart so that he could effect penetration.

Although the girls and their mother related what they had seen him do to others, each denied that they themselves had actually been penetrated. Moreover, the only member of the community willing to give evidence was a patient in a tuberculosis sanatorium at some distance from the community at the time of the investigation. Although Hiram's brother and his wife talked to the neighbor about Hiram, they refused to say anything to the police and, when the neighbor asked Bernice why she had not reported her father's acts, Bernice ignored her completely. The community complained to school officials that Hiram threatened people with death by witchcraft, that they were terrorized and unable to do anything. The evidence of Hiram's evil power was overwhelming; he was a Flintway singer, was known to have committed incest, and one of his granddaughters was retarded.

The tribal police believed the FBI would not accept the case for federal prosecution because the witnesses were not forthcoming, and the tribal court could not impose a sentence that would keep Hiram out of the community for any length of time. Hiram continued to live in the community for another fifteen years until, at the age of eighty-eight, he died from exposure after becoming lost in a blizzard. The body was found several days after the storm cleared and was buried where it lay.

Hiram's sexual impulses were hostile and aimed at females whom he could control. His ability to sustain sexual relations with his daughter and stepdaughter for years after they reached maturity is not common among those who commit incest and suggests that his hostility and need to control were derived from something more than the sexual immaturity of the pedophile or the unresolved Oedipal feelings of the incest offender.

Why the social controls available to the community did not function effectively needs explication. The legal system was powerless to act because members of the community refused to testify in court. Witch killing is justifiable in the eyes of traditional Navajos, but today is rare because the courts do not recognize witchcraft's existence and would prosecute the witch killer for murder. Nevertheless, there are instances of "justifiable homicide" committed by individuals who take matters into their own hands. We have direct knowledge of a case which the tribal police neither investigated nor made note of in their records despite the fact they had been called on to remove the body. Hiram was one of those rare individuals who, undeterred by the threat of being accused of witchcraft, openly accepted the role and used it to his own advantage. Given these circumstances, no one had the courage to kill him.

More recently, a woman accused her husband of seducing his stepdaughter. Although this was never proven, his behavior toward his stepdaughter had become very seductive and, at the same time, very authoritarian as he sought to control every area of her life. The marriage dissolved, and the husband left the community. As in Hiram's case, the need to dominate the female was as important as the sexual attraction.

We believe that father-daughter incest occurred with about as much frequency as sibling incest, that it was as abhorred and feared, and that its consequences were as disruptive. But why, if this is so, was it never thought to be the cause of an important disease? Father-daughter incest is associated with Coyote in the archetypal "trickster marries his daughter" myth found among most of the hunting tribes of western North America. This myth continues to exist among the Navajos but is not contained in the origin legends of any of the healing ceremonies. We believe that, during the period when Navajo religion was "Puebloized," the association of incest with Coyote was de-emphasized.

To illustrate the point, let us look briefly at how Coyote and incest are positioned in Navajo mythology. The creation myth as we know it is told according to the Blessingway tradition. It tells of the emergence from the underworlds and is the "main stalk" from which the myths of all the healing ceremonies branch off. The origin of witchcraft, so intimately associated with Coyote in the healing chants, is here attributed to First Man and First Woman. First Woman witches her own children, who later marry each other and learn witchcraft. There is some suggestion that First Man and First Woman are also siblings: "Mother Earth and Father Sky teach their children, First Man and First Woman, the Big Witch Ceremony, after which 'they lived there together,' i.e., as man and wife" (K. Spencer, 1947:107). The only marriage regula-

tions mentioned are those prohibiting marriage between siblings
and with a person of one's own clan. And no reference is made to
the preferred marriages of the pastoral period such as the sororate,
the levirate, marriage to a woman and her daughter, or the tendency for a group of siblings to marry other groups of siblings (K.
Spencer 1947:33–34). Even the account of Coyote's excesses during the separation of the sexes only mentions that he copulates
with his sisters.

Coyote's association with death and witchcraft is preserved
in the myths of the healing chants, but the story of Coyote's
witchcraft is most often that of the hero who is transformed by
Coyote so that the latter can seduce the hero's wives. The story
of Coyote's seduction of his daughter's is one of a series of tales
about "Trotting Coyote" (Haile 1984:47–52; Hill and Hill
1945; Matthews 1885). It is not found in Evilway but is included as a minor motif in some versions of Mountainway (Wyman 1975:148–51). A number of sings contain the "witch
father-in-law" theme, however (K. Spencer 1957:28–29). In
these stories, the hero comes upon a family, consisting of a
father, mother, and daughter, living off by themselves. Although the hero is greeted as a son-in-law, it transpires that the
father is a witch, living incestously with his daughter, who
tries to destroy him. Thus, the picture of family isolation, incest, and witchcraft is clearly outlined, even though Coyote is
not directly involved. Nevertheless, when we asked the singer
who told us about Mothway why only Coyote had the medicines for incest, he mentioned Coyote's incest with his daughter. Although siblings who commit incest are not accused of
witchcraft despite the prominence of the association in myth,
ceremonialists with epileptic children are reluctant to have
sings performed for them or to bring them to medical attention
because, we believe, they fear witchcraft accusations and suspicions of having committed incest.

Our cases of frenzy witchcraft are puzzling. We have re-
marked that the myth comes from Zuni where, at least until
the late nineteenth century, love magic was thought to cause
seizures and was punishable by death. Today, however, the practice appears to have died out entirely, and we found no cases of
seizures attributed to this form of witchcraft. Among the West-

ern Apaches practitioners of love magic were never thought to be real witches, and it appears not to have been a real problem. The Navajos have retained the beliefs, the mythology, and the healing ceremony until very recently. Yet none of the people said to have been witched in this manner and treated with Frenzy-witchcraftway were thought to have been victimized by a man who wished to seduce them. Instead the stories were of witchery with intent to kill. Disturbed father-daughter relationships appeared in a variety of ways. First, of course, is the fact that in popular belief frenzy witchcraft is practiced by older men who wish to seduce young women. Among our cases were several women who accused their fathers or grandfathers of trying to witch them, others who were rebelling against authoritarian and controlling fathers, and one who exhibited an incestuous attraction for her father at the same time she was trying to free herself from him. None of the cases of frenzy witchcraft involved actual father-daughter incest. Nevertheless, in some vague manner, this form of witchcraft, and the seizures it is thought to produce, seem to be associated with father-daughter incest.

Concluding Remarks

Our understanding of the meaning that seizures and incest have in Navajo culture was arrived at by emphasizing the historical development of Navajo religion and proposing that attitudes and beliefs about incest were shaped by changing economic and social conditions. Where others have emphasized two historical periods, the Pueblo and pre-Pueblo, we have insisted on the importance of the pastoral period which lasted from the late eighteenth to the early twentieth century. Although the myth symbols and motifs were borrowed from the Pueblos, they retained their immediacy because they were updated to the social environment that emerged during these years. We have raised the possibility that the Apaches were also concerned about incest because they seem to have a personality configuration very similar to that of the Navajos. If this is so, the differences in their beliefs about incest, its causes and consequences, can only be explained by historical events that

were experienced only by the Navajos. In effect, while the involvement with incest may possibly be equally intense among
the two groups, the cultural elements used to express this concern are very different.

The reader will have discerned that Kaplan's notion of a general Navajo predisposition to ego abdication has neither been
confirmed nor denied. We have shown that Navajos do not generally attribute disease to possession or to soul loss as he believed, although they may have done so prior to their arrival in
the Southwest. We have also seen that the prevalence of hysterical disease may not be higher among the Navajos than it is
in the general population and that the psychological problems
of Navajo epileptics account for the difference in the rates of
hysteria among Navajos and Pueblos. These findings suggest
that we are not dealing with an aspect of the basic personality
but with the effects of a specific cultural belief on a limited
number of individuals who are so unfortunate as to suffer from
epilepsy. On the other hand, Boyer's characterization of Apache
personality configuration is so similar to that of the Navajos
that we cannot dismiss out of hand the idea that the hysterical
aspects of Apache personality are present among the Navajos
also. We would like to know, for example, whether a survey of
hand tremblers would reveal that many have hysterical personalities.

It may already be too late to pursue these and other questions
further, however. The stock reduction programs of the 1930s
and 1940s effectively destroyed the Navajos' pastoral adapta-
tion. Those who were born and reared in that culture are now
old, their numbers rapidly dwindling. The social and economic
environment has changed drastically since 1940. Stockraising
provides for less than 5 percent of total income in the area.
Isolation has been decreased by improved transportation, population growth, and the fact that almost all children are in
school. Few Navajo infants are breast-fed today, and demand
feeding is less prevalent now that many young mothers have
jobs. Some Navajos are consciously rejecting traditional beliefs, others are growing up in environments that preclude
learning and experiencing them, with the result that they lose
their emotional content. Today a young man may be taught
that ghosts cause illness, but he will not experience death in

the home with any frequency and he will have little or no cause to handle a corpse, abandon a hogan, or perform a traditional burial.[7] How then can the "awe" of dangerous forces be internalized?

Nor will it be an easy task to study asymptomatic incest offenders to determine what ceremonial treatments are prescribed for them. Already in the 1960s, Mothway and Coyoteway according to its Evil side were extinct. The ten Frenzywitchcraftway singers we identified in the western Navajo reservation have all died, and there has been no one to take their places. A complete nine-night performance of Mountainway has not been performed in the area for over fifteen years and soon it too may become moribund. Henderson (1982) has shown how rapidly the number of ceremonialists has declined in the area. Today, the majority of singers know the less dangerous sings, especially Blessingway.

Navajo religion will not die but will collapse upon itself. Blessingway, combined with a few songs from one of the exorcistic sings, will become the typical "traditional" cure. Already medical entrepreneurs are providing for patients who want a "traditional" ceremony but who cannot pay for a performance lasting more than a few hours. Hand tremblers have learned some Blessingway prayers and some songs from some of the more common curing ceremonies, thus combining diagnostic skills with short curing rituals. This is a first step in the transformation of a self-contained healing system into folk medicine.

This book has been concerned almost exclusively with pain and suffering, little attention being paid to healing and happiness. This is almost inevitable when the aim of the research is to learn more about a disease and those afflicted with it. Many Navajos believe that paying as much attention as we have to dangerous things is itself dangerous, and the singers who instructed us were emphatic in their insistence that human life would be impossible without the "good" side. Lest there be any misunderstanding on this point, our aim in writing this book has been to increase our knowledge about seizures in Navajo culture and not to accord them or the concept of *hóchǫ́ǫ́* in which they are embedded precedence over the other side of Navajo religion and healing.

Notes

1. Introduction

1. Pueblitos are sites containing small Pueblo style structures varying in number from one to many, with associated hogans, towers, and defensive walls.

2. The Healing Tradition

1. We are indebted to David Shaul and Emory Sekaquaptewa for helping us trace the linguistic parallels and Hopi usages of these two terms.

2. For a more complete discussion of Pueblo shamanism, see Levy (in press). For information on the distribution of bear shamans, refer to Jorgensen (1980:294–95).

3. For such states among the Tewas, see Laski (1958:96–97, 103–7, 110–13, 115, notes 151–56). For Isleta, see Parsons (1930:193–466, pp. 248, 285, 444). For the Keresans, see White (1930:107, 110, 121), and Lange (1968:233, 236). For Zuni, see Bunzel (1932a:489), and Stevenson (1904:478, 494, 495, 500, 502, 503, 563).

4. The two shaman societies were the *poshwimpkya* and the *yayatu*. The former cured individuals suffering from conditions caused by witchcraft, employed the sucking cure, and used datura to induce trance states. The *yayatu* shamans used the extraordinary powers of the Keresan Bear shamans to travel great distances in an instant, to fly, and to survive fire and falls from cliffs. They were charged with the task of protecting the community from such disasters as famine and drought and were known for public exhibitions of their powers. Not only were trance states utilized by the shamans, but datura was used to induce them. It is believed that these societies were adopted as recently as the eighteenth century and, according to the Hopis, did not last very long, ostensibly because the rigors of fasting and continence imposed on their members were too onerous. These shamans were not thought to derive their power from the bear, however, and the bear was not considered one of the great healing animals. Although the Hopis experimented with these imported societies, they refused to allow the bear, the most potent symbol of the power of the individual shaman, to occupy an important position in the cosmology. The last surviving members of the *poshwimpkya* were known to have performed sucking cures and to have utilized shaman-

istic trance states. Aside from these individuals, however, the majority of Hopi curers look more like charismatic healers than shamans. See Beaglehole and Beaglehole (1935:9–10), A.F. Whiting (1939:31, 89), and Stephen (1969:xii, x, xviii, 460, 1007–8).

5. What has been recorded may be found in Hill (1936 and 1938).

6. The Navajos do not rely on the solstitial division of the year but define winter as the period between the first and last frost.

7. Also considered "dangerous" are Mothway, Frenzy-witchcraft-way, Coyoteway, and Mountainway. See, for example, Kluckhohn (1962:231) for a statement concerning the dangerous aspects of Frenzy-witchcraftway and the belief that, like Evilway, it had its origins before the emergence.

3. Beliefs About Seizures

1. In 1962 and 1963, Levy and Parker interviewed all mental patients admitted to the Tuba City Hospital prior to their transfer to Phoenix for psychiatric evaluation.

2. This woman became very distraught during the interview and many of the details of the ceremonial procedure were provided by her 65-year-old daughter, who had learned of the episode from her aunt who had pulled the informant from the fire and had been present at the ceremony.

3. The girls are referred to as "non-sunlight-struck maidens" who have been sequestered in a subterranean chamber to keep them from the sun's rays. The reference is to virginity because the girls have been shielded from the fertilizing rays of the sun.

4. This ceremony is said to cure all sorts of madness. It contains the story of "Changing Bear Maiden," which tells of how Coyote married the Bear Maiden and taught her all his evil witchery. In effect, the dangerous qualities of bears are derived from Coyote.

5. Pueblo and Navajo clans are grouped into "phratries" (or clan groups), which are also exogamous. Thus, although there are more than sixty Navajo clans, there are only nine clan groups.

6. Marriage always involves some conflict of loyalties. In order to reduce such conflicts, people prefer to make alliances with families already related to them in some way. In societies with unilineal descent, a preference for marriage into father's clan creates alliances between the same kin groups in succeeding generations.

7. Scholars are not agreed on whether the Navajos developed matrilineal descent before or after their arrival in the Southwest. Driver and Massey, and Murdock, for example, believe that, like most North

American hunting and gathering groups, the Navajos had bilateral descent and only began to develop matrilineality after a period of contact with various Pueblo groups and the attendant adoption of agriculture. According to Dyen and Aberle, however, the Navajos and Apaches were most probably matrilineal when they entered the Southwest. See Driver and Massey (1957), Dyen and Aberle (1975), and Murdock (1949, 1955:85-97).

8. For a more complete discussion of these marriage restrictions, see Aberle (1980:105-43).

4. The Epidemiology of Seizures and Pseudoseizures

1. For a more complete, nontechnical discussion of epilepsy than is presented here, see Lechtenberg (1984). An up-to-date review of the syndrome is provided in Epilepsy Foundation of America (1981).

2. For an unusually lucid account of Freud's final thoughts on hysteria, see Nemiah (1967).

3. The Indian Health Service estimate of the Navajo population of the Tuba City Service Unit on December 31, 1976, is 10,000 and for the resident Tewa population, 2,500. The estimate of the Hopi population on the reservation and in the village of Moenkopi in 1975 was 6,054. We used an annual population increase of 1.75 percent to arrive at a prevalence day estimate of 6,200. The Bureau of Indian Affairs estimate of the Zuni population for December 1976 is 6,300 and includes those Zunis temporarily away from the reservation.

4. In addition to those in residence during the entire five-year period, we included (a) children away at school who returned home for summer vacations; (b) those reared on the reservation who had left to take jobs elsewhere who were not in residence on prevalence day if they had been on reservation for three of the five previous years; (c) those who had taken jobs away from the reservation but were in residence on prevalence day if they had been on the reservation for the prior twelve months.

5. Because Indian populations are considerably younger than the general population, rates have been age-adjusted. Initially, the Hopi rate was 6.9 but, after an adjustment was made to allow for a number of missing charts, the revised rate was 8.0.

6. Dr. Charles North has calculated equally high rates of *Haemophilus influenza* meningitis among the Hopi (personal communication). For North American Indian rates generally, see Feldman, Koehler, and Fraser (1976).

5. Navajo Diagnosis and Treatment

1. 103 individuals were members of a rural extended kin group living about 25 miles from the Tuba City hospital. Another 106 people were living in households randomly selected from a census of households south of the Tuba City trading post. This latter group represents approximately a third of what was known as the South Tuba community. Although the most acculturated and wage-work-oriented settlement in the Service Unit at that time, the average number of sings performed per capita did not differ among the two groups.

2. The ritual is used by people who dream of sexual intercourse or who have itching in the genital regions or difficulty urinating. The *vagina dentata* monster of the origin myth is said to be the cause of these disorders. In Mountainway this monster is identified as a bear and one of the figurines used in the ritual is said to be the vagina of Changing Bear Maiden. See Haile (1947:47–57).

3. Coyoteway is one of the Holyway chants that use masked gods. Its myth identifies Coyote as the creator of corn. Luckert believes it to have been derived from Pueblo traditions. We do not believe that the Whirling Coyote ritual or the Rabid Dog songs come from the Coyoteway recorded by Luckert and others but are from an older, long extinct sing once part of the Evilway group of chants. The only singer we found who knew these rituals claimed they were not a part of Coyoteway but refused to say more on the subject. This man was a Frenzy-witchcraftway singer. See Luckert (1979).

4. In many myths Coyote is discovered because of the smell of his urine, which he is not able to disguise even when he transforms himself into other forms. The informants may be stretching a point to claim that Coyote urinated everywhere because of seizures, however.

5. See Spencer (1957) for a review of the myth motifs of the healing ceremonies.

6. A comprehensive discussion of this may be found in Witherspoon (1977:13–62).

6. Hand Trembling

1. See the discussion in Lewis (1971:179–80).

9. Ambivalence, Anxiety, and Incest

1. "Shared fathers' clan" is a term used to refer to marriage between individuals whose fathers belong to the same clan.

2. The similarity of Navajo and Apache personality configurations will be commented upon below. Whether, as the Kaska data might

suggest, Athabascans in general are concerned about incest is a question we cannot comment upon here. Hippler, Boyer, and Boyer (1976) believe that modern Athabascans everywhere have a common basic personality which developed in response to the harsh subarctic environment and which has persisted despite the migrations and changes experienced by the southern groups.

3. An excellent discussion of the various social controls used to resolve conflicts in a Navajo community is provided by Shepardson and Hammond (1970:128–56).

4. The mother's sisters' children. Residence was matrilocal in most instances, so that children of a mother's brother or of a father's siblings would rarely be part of the camp. Mother's sister's children belong to the same clan and are referred to by the same terms used for one's own brothers and sisters.

5. For a discussion and references, see Spencer (1947:24–26).

6. We are indebted to Mary Shepardson for bringing this case to our attention and for making her notes available to us.

7. For a discussion of some of these changes, see Levy (1978:397–405).

Bibliography

ABERLE, DAVID F.
1961 "Navaho." In *Matrilineal Kinship*, edited by David M. Schneider and Kathleen Gough, 96–201. Berkeley: University of California Press.
1980 "Navajo Exogamic Rules and Preferred Marriages." In *The Versatility of Kinship: Essays Presented to Harry W. Basehart*, edited by Linda S. Cordell and Stephen Beckerman, 105–43. New York: Academic Press.

ABSE, D. WILFRED
1950 *The Diagnosis of Hysteria*. Bristol: Wright.
1959 "Hysteria." In *American Handbook of Psychiatry*, edited by Silvano Arieti, 272–91. New York: Basic Books.

AITKEN, BARBARA (FEIRE-MARRECO)
1930 "Temperament in Native American Religion." *Journal of the Royal Anthropological Institute of Great Britain and Ireland*, 60:363–87.

AMERICAN PSYCHIATRIC ASSOCIATION
1980 *Diagnostic and Statistical Manual of Mental Disorders*. 3rd ed. Washington: APA.

BASSO, KEITH H.
1969 *Western Apache Witchcraft*, University of Arizona Anthropological Paper 15. Tucson: University of Arizona Press.

BEAGLEHOLE, ERNEST, AND PEARL BEAGLEHOLE
1935 *Hopi of the Second Mesa*. Memoir of the American Anthropological Association 44. Menasha, Wisconsin: American Anthropological Association.

BENEDICT, PAUL K.
1958 "Socio-Cultural Factors in Schizophrenia." In *Schizophrenia: A Review of the Syndrome*, edited by Leopold Bellak, 694–729. New York: Logos Press.

BENEDICT, RUTH
1960 *Patterns of Culture*. 1934. Reprint. New York: Mentor.

BENNETT, JOHN H.
1946 "The Integration of Pueblo Culture: A Question of Values." *Southwestern Journal of Anthropology*. 2:361–74.

BOYER, L. BRYCE
1979 *Childhood and Folklore: A Psychoanalytic Study of Apache Personality*. New York: The Library of Psychological Anthropology.

BOYER, L. BRYCE, B. KLOPFER, F. B. BRAWER, AND H. KAWAI
1964 "Comparisons of Shamans and Pseudoshamans of the Apaches of the Mescalero Indian Reservation: A Rorschach Study." *Journal of Projective Techniques.* 28:173–80.

BRANDT, RICHARD B.
1954 *Hopi Ethics: A Theoretical Analysis.* Chicago: University of Chicago Press.

BREUER, JOSEF, AND SIGMUND FREUD
1937 *Studies on Hysteria.* 1895. Reprint. Boston: Nervous and Mental Disease Publishing Co.

BRUGGE, DAVID M.
1963 *Navajo Pottery and Ethnohistory.* Window Rock: Navajoland Publications, Navajo Tribal Museum.
1983 "Navajo History and Prehistory to 1850." In *Handbook of North American Indians, 10, Southwest,* edited by Alfonso Ortiz, 489–501. Washington, D.C.: Smithsonian Institution.

BUNZEL, RUTH
1932a "Introduction to Zuni Ceremonialism." U.S. Bureau of Ethnology *Annual Report* 47:467–544.
1932b "Zuni Katcinas." U.S. Bureau of Ethnology *Annual Report* 47:837–1086.

CARROLL, MICHAEL P.
1984 "The Trickster-Father Feigns Death and Commits Incest:
/85 Some Methodological Contributions to the Study of Myth." *Behavior Science Research* 19:24–57.

COULEHAN, JOHN L. ET AL.
1976 "Bacterial Meningitis in Navajo Indians." *Public Health Reports.* 91:464–68.
1981 "Haemophilus Influenza and Other Bacterial Meningitis Among Navajo Indians: 1974–1980." Unpublished ms.

CUSHING, FRANK H.
1896 "Outlines of Zuni Creation Myths." U.S. Bureau of American Ethnology *Annual Report* 13:321–447.

DONGIER, S.
1959 "Statistical Study of Clinical and Electroencephalographic Manifestations of 536 Psychotic Episodes Occurring in 516 Epileptics Between Clinical Seizures." *Epilepsia,* 1:117–42.

DRIVER, HAROLD E., AND WILLIAM C. MASSEY
1957 *Comparative Studies of North American Indians.* American Philosophical Society, Transactions, n.s., vol. 476, pt.2.

DUBE, K. C., AND NARENDER KUMAR
1974 "An Epidemiological Study of Hysteria." *Journal of Biosocial Sciences.* 6:401–05.

DYEN, ISIDORE AND DAVID F. ABERLE
1975 *Lexical Reconstruction: The Case of the Proto-Athabascan Kinship System.* London: Cambridge University Press.

DYK, WALTER
1947 *A Navaho Autobiography.* New York: Viking Funds Publications in Anthropology, 8.

EPILEPSY FOUNDATION OF AMERICA
1981 *How to Recognize and Classify Seizures.* Landover, Maryland: The Epilepsy Foundation of America.

FELDMAN, R. A., R. E. KOEHLER, AND D. W. FRASER
1976 "Race Specific Differences in Bacterial Meningitis Deaths in the United States, 1962–1968." *American Journal of Public Health.* 66:392–96.

FISHLER, STANLEY A.
1953 *In the Beginning: A Navajo Creation Myth.* Salt Lake City: University of Utah, Department of Anthropology Paper, 13.

FOULKS, EDWARD F.
1972 *The Arctic Hysterias of the North Alaskan Eskimo. Anthropological Studies, 10.* Menasha, Wisconsin: American Anthropological Association.

FRANCISCAN FATHERS, THE
1910 *Ethnologic Dictionary of the Navaho Language.* St. Michaels, Arizona: The Franciscan Fathers.

FRAZER, JAMES, SIR
1922 *The Golden Bough* (abridged). New York: Macmillan.

GOODWIN, GRENVILLE
1969 *The Social Organization of the Western Apache.* Tucson: University of Arizona Press.

GOUGH, KATHLEEN
1961 "Variation in Preferential Marriage Forms." In *Matrilineal Kinship,* edited by David M. Schneider and Kathleen Gough, 614–30. Berkeley: University of California Press.

GUBSER, N.
1965 *Nunemiut Eskimos: Hunters of Caribou.* New Haven: Yale University Press.

HAILE, BERARD
1947 *Navaho Sacrificial Figurines.* Chicago: University of Chicago Press.

1950   *Legend of the Ghostway Ritual in the Male Branch of Shootingway and Suckingway in its Legend and Practice.* St. Michaels, Arizona: St. Michaels Press.

1978   *Love Magic and Butterfly People: The Slim Curley Version of the Ajitee and Mothway Myths.* Edited by Karl W. Luckert. Flagstaff: Museum of Northern Arizona Press.

1984   *Navajo Coyote Tales: The Curley Tó Ahedliinii Version.* Edited by Karl W. Luckert. Lincoln: University of Nebraska Press.

HALLIDAY, A. M. AND A. A. MASON
1963   "The Effects of Hypnotic Anaesthesia on Cortical Responses." *Journal of Neurology, Neurosurgery and Psychiatry,* 9:300–12.

HARVEY, YOUNGSOOK KIM
1979   *Six Korean Women: The Socialization of Shamans.* St. Paul. West Publishing Co.

HAUSER, W. ALLEN AND LEONARD T. KURLAND
1975   "The Epidemiology of Epilepsy in Rochester, Minnesota, 1935 through 1967." *Epilepsia* 16:1–66.

HENDERSON, ERIC B.
1982   "Kaibeto Plateau Ceremonialists, 1860–1980." In *Navajo Religion and Culture: Selected Views. Papers in Honor of Leland C. Wyman,* edited by David M. Brugge and Charlotte J. Frisbie, 164–75. Santa Fé: Museum of New Mexico Press.

HILL, W. W.
1936   *Navaho Warfare,* New Haven: Yale University Publications in Anthropology, 5.

1938   *The Agricultural and Hunting Methods of the Navaho Indians.* New Haven: Yale University Publications in Anthropology, 18.

HILL, W. W. AND DOROTHY HILL
1945   "Navaho Coyote Tales and Their Position in the Southern Athabascan Group." *Journal of American Folklore* 58:335–337.

HIPPLER, ARTHUR E., L. BRYCE BOYER, AND RUTH M. BOYER
1976   "The Subarctic Athabascans of Canada: The Ecological Grounding of Certain Cultural Personality Characteristics." *The Psychoanalytic Study of Society* 7:293–329.

HOEBEL, E. ADAMSON
1940   *The Political Organization and Law-Ways of the Comanche Indians. American Anthropological Association Memoir 54.*

Menasha, Wisconsin: American Anthropological Association.

HONIGMAN, JOHN J.
1954 *The Kaska Indians: An Ethnographic Reconstruction.* Yale University Publications in Anthropology, 51.

JOHNSON, D. M.
1945 "The Phantom Anesthetist of Mattoon: A Field Study of Mass Hysteria." *Journal of Abnormal and Social Psychology* 40:175–86.

JONES, J. A.
1964 "Rio Grande Pueblo Albinism." *American Journal of Physical Anthropology* 22:265–74.

JORGENSEN, JOSEPH G.
1980 *Western Indians: Comparative Environments, Languages, and Cultures of 172 Western American Indian Tribes.* San Francisco: W. H. Freeman and Co.

KAPLAN, BERT AND DALE JOHNSON
1964 "The Social Meaning of Navaho Psychopathology and Psychotherapy." In *Magic, Faith, and Healing: Studies in Primitive Psychiatry Today*, edited by Ari Kiev, 203–29. London: The Free Press of Glencoe, Collier Macmillan, Ltd.

KLUCKHOHN, CLYDE
1962 *Navaho Witchcraft.* 2d ed. Boston: Beacon Press.

KNIGHT, J. A., T. I. FRIEDMAN AND J. SULLIANTI
1965 "Epidemic Hysteria: A Field Study." *American Journal of Public Health* 55:858–65.

KRETSCHMER, ERNEST
1926 *Hysteria.* New York: Nervous and Mental Disease Publishing Co.

KROEBER, ALFRED L.
1952 *The Nature of Culture.* Chicago: University of Chicago Press.

KSENOFONTOV, G. V.
1955 *Schamengeschichten aus Siberien.* 2d ed. Munich: Otto Wilhelm Barth Verlag.

KURLAND, LEONARD T., JOHN F. KURTZKE AND IRVING D. GOLDBERG
1973 *Epidemiology of Neurologic and Sense Organ Disorders.* Cambridge: Harvard University Press.

LAMPHERE, LOUISE
1983 "Southwestern Ceremonialism." In *Handbook of North American Indians, 11, Southwest*, edited by Alfonso Ortiz, 743–63. Washington: Smithsonian Institution.

LANDAR, HERBERT
1967   "The Language of Pain in Navajo Culture." In *Studies in Southwestern Linguistics: Meaning and History in the Languages of the American Southwest*, edited by Del Hymes and William E. Bittle, 119–44. The Hague: Mouton and Co.

LANGE, CHARLES H.
1968   *Cochiti: A New Mexico Pueblo Past and Present.* 2d ed., Carbondale: Southern Illinois University Press.

LASKI, VERA
1958   *Seeking Life.* Philadelphia: American Folklore Society Memoir, 50.

LEBRA, WILLIAM B.
1969   "Shaman and Client in Okinawa." In *Mental Health Research in Asia and the Pacific*, edited by William Caudill and T. Y. Lin, 216–22. Honolulu: East-West Center Press.

LECHTENBERG, RICHARD
1984   *Epilepsy and the Family.* Cambridge: Harvard University Press.

LEIGHTON, DOROTHEA C., AND CLYDE KLUCKHOHN
1947   *Children of the People.* Cambridge: Harvard University Press.

LEIGHTON, DOROTHEA C., JOHN S. HARDING, DAVID B. MACKLIN, ALLISTER MACMILLAN, AND ALEXANDER H. LEIGHTON
1963   *The Character of Danger.* New York: Basic Books.

LEMKAU, PAUL V., AND GUIDO M. CROCETTI
1958   "Vital Statistics of Schizophrenia." In *Schizophrenia: A Review of the Syndrome*, edited by Leopold Bellak, 64–81. New York: Logos Pres'

LÉVI-STRAUSS, CLAUDE
1963   *Structural Anthropology.* New York: Basic Books.

LEVY, JERROLD E.
1965   "Navajo Suicide." *Human Organization* 24:308–18.
1978   "Changing Burial Practices of the Western Navajo: A Consideration of the Relationship Between Attitudes and Behavior." *American Indian Quarterly* 4:397–405.
1983   "Traditional Navajo Health Beliefs and Practices." In *Disease Change and the Role of Medicine: The Navajo Experience*, edited by Stephen J. Kunitz, 118–45. Berkely: University of California Press.
In   "Hopi Shamanism: A Reappraisal." In *Essays in Honor of*
press   *Fred Eggan*, edited by Alfonso Ortiz and Ray deMallie. Chicago: University of Chicago Press.

LEVY, JERROLD E., AND STEPHEN J. KUNITZ
1971   "Indian Reservations, Anomie, and Social Pathologies."
       Southwestern Journal of Anthropology 27:97–128.
1974   Indian Drinking: Navajo Practices and Anglo-American
       Theories. New York: John Wiley and Sons.
1986   "Depression among Elderly Navajos." Paper presented at the
       joint meeting of the Society for Medical Anthropology and
       the British Medical Anthropology Society, New Hall,
       Cambridge University, Cambridge, England, June 30–July 3,
       1986.
LEVY, JERROLD E., STEPHEN J. KUNITZ, AND ERIC B. HENDERSON
In   "Hopi Deviance in Historical and Epidemiological Perspec-
press tive." In Themes in Ethnology and Culture History: Essays
       in Honor of David F. Aberle, edited by Joseph G. Jorgensen
       and Leland Donald. Berkeley: Folklore Institute Press.
LEVY, JERROLD E., RAYMOND NEUTRA, AND DENNIS PARKER
1979   "Life Careers of Navajo Epileptics." Social Science and Med-
       icine 13B:53–66.
LEWIS, I. M.
1971   Ecstatic Religion: An Anthropological Study of Spirit Posses-
       sion and Shamanism. Middlesex: Penguin Books.
LEWIS, W. C., AND M. BERMAN
1965   "Studies of Conversion Hysteria. I. Operational Study of Di-
       agnoses." Archives of General Psychiatry 13:274–82.
LINTON, RALPH
1956   Culture and Mental Disorders. Springfield, Illinois: Charles
       C. Thomas.
LJUNBERG, LENNART
1957   "Hysteria: A Clinical, Prognostic, and Genetic Study." Acta
       Psychiatrica Scandinavia 32, Supplement 112.
LLEWELLYN, KARL N., AND E. ADAMSON HOEBEL
1941   The Cheyenne Way: Conflict and Case Law in Primitive Ju-
       risprudence. Norman: University of Oklahoma Press.
LOWIE, ROBERT H.
1961   Primitive Society. New York: Harper and Brothers.
LUCKERT, KARL W.
1975   The Navajo Hunter Tradition. Tucson: University of Ari-
       zona Press.
1978   A Navajo Bringing Home Ceremony: The Claus Chee Sonny
       Version of Deerway Ajiłee. Flagstaff: Museum of Northern
       Arizona Press.

1979   *Coyoteway: A Navajo Holyway Healing Ceremonial.* Tucson: University of Arizona Press.
1981   "Editor's Introduction." In *Upward Moving and Emergence Way: The Gishen Biye' Version*, edited by Berard Haile, i–xv. Lincoln: University of Nebraska Press.

MASTERS, R. E. L.
1963   *Patterns of Incest: A Psycho-Social Study of Incest Based on Clinical and Historic Data.* New York: Julian Press.

MATTHEWS, WASHINGTON
1885   "The Origin of the Utes, a Navaho Myth." *American Antiquarian and Oriental Journal* 7:271–73.
1887   "The Mountain Chant: A Navaho Ceremony." U.S. Bureau of American Ethnology *Annual Report* 5:379–467.

MCKEGNY, F. P.
1967   "The Incidence and Characteristics of Patients with Conversion Reactions. I. A. General Consultation Service Sample." *American Journal of Psychiatry* 124:542–45.

MITCHELL, FRANK
1978   *Navajo Blessingway Singer: The Autobiography of Frank Mitchell, 1881–1967.* Edited by Charlotte Frisbie and David P. McAllester. Tucson: University of Arizona Press.

MURDOCK, GEORGE P.
1949   *Social Structure.* New York: Macmillan.
1955   "North American Social Organization." *Davidson Journal of Anthropology* 1:85–97.

MURPHY, H. B. M.
1976   "Notes for a Theory on Latah." In *Culture Bound Syndromes*, edited by William Lebra, 3–21. Honolulu: University Press of Hawaii.

MURPHY, JANE M.
1964   "Psychotherapeutic Aspects of Shamanism on St. Lawrence Island." In *Magic, Faith, and Healing: Studies in Primitive Psychiatry Today*, edited by Ari Kiev, 53–83. London: The Free Press of Glencoe, Collier Macmillan Ltd.

NEMIA, JOHN C.
1967   "Conversion Reaction." In *Comprehensive Textbook of Psychiatry*, edited by Alfred M. Freedman and Harold I. Kaplan, 870–84. Baltimore: Williams and Wilkins.

O'BRYAN, AILEEN
1956   *The Diné: Origin Myths of the Navajos Indians.* U.S. Bureau of American Ethnology Bulletin, 163.

OPLER, MORRIS EDWARD
1938   "Ethnological Notes." In *Chiricahua and Mescalero Apache*

Texts, edited by Harry Hoijer, 141–56, 214–19. Chicago: University of Chicago Press.

1965   *An Apache Life-Way: The Economic, Social, and Religious Institutions of the Chiricahua Indians*. New York: Cooper Square Publishers.

ORNE, M.T.
1959   "The Nature of Hypnosis: Artifact and Essence." *Journal of Abnormal and Social Psychology* 58:277–99.

PARSONS, ELSIE CLEWS
1930   "Isleta." U.S. Bureau of American Ethnology *Annual Report* 47:193–466.
1974   *Pueblo Indian Religion*. 4 vols. 1939. Reprint. Chicago: University of Chicago Press.

PRICE-WILLIAMS, DOUGLAS R.
1975   *Explorations in Cross-Cultural Psychology*. San Francisco: Chandler and Sharp.

RADIN, PAUL
1972   *The Trickster: A Study in American Indian Mythology*. (1st published 1956), New York: Schocken Books.

REICHARD, GLADYS
1963   *Navaho Religion: A Study of Symbolism*. 2d ed., New York: Pantheon Books.

SASAKI, YUJI
1969   "Psychiatric Study of the Shaman in Japan." In *Mental Health Research in Asia and the Pacific*, edited by William Caudill and T. Y. Lin, 223–41. Honolulu: East-West Center Press.

SCHMERLA, HENRIETTA
1931   "Trickster Marries His Daughter." *Journal of American Folklore* 44:196–207.

SCHULER, E. A., AND V. J. A. PRENTON
1943   "A Recent Epidemic of Hysteria in a Louisiana High School." *Journal of Social Psychology* 17:221–35.

SHEPARDSON, MARY, AND BLODWEN HAMMOND
1970   *The Navajo Mountain Community: Social Organization and Kinship Terminology*. Berkeley: University of California Press.

SILVERMAN, J.
1967   "Shamans and Acute Schizophrenia." *American Anthropologist* 69:21–31.

SON OF OLD MAN HAT
1967   *Son of Old Man Hat: A Navaho Autobiography*. Recorded by Walter Dyk, 2d ed. Lincoln: University of Nebraska Press.

SPENCER, KATHERINE
1947   *Reflections of Social Life in the Navaho Creation Myth.* Albuquerque: University of New Mexico Press.
1957   *Mythology and Values: An Analysis of Navaho Chantway Myths.* Philadelphia: American Folklore Society.

SPENCER, ROBERT F.
1959   *The North Alaskan Eskimo.* U.S. Bureau of American Ethnology Bulletin, 171.

SPUHLER, JAMES N., AND CLYDE KLUCKHOHN
1953   "Inbreeding Coefficients of the Ramah Navaho Population." *Human Biology* 25:295–317.

STEFANSSON, J. G., J. A. MESSINA, AND S. MEYEROWITZ
1976   "Hysterical Neurosis, Conversion Type: Clinical and Epidemiological Considerations." *Acta Psychiatrica Scandinavia* 53:119–38.

STEPHEN, ALEXANDER M.
1929   "Hopi Tales." *Journal of American Folklore* 42 (163):1–72.
1969   *Hopi Journal of Alexander M. Stephen.* 2d ed., edited by Elsie Clews Parsons. New York: AMS Press.

STEVENSON, MATILDA COX
1904   "The Zuni Indians." U.S. Bureau of American Ethnology, *Annual Report* 23:1–634.

STEWARD, JULIAN H.
1933   *Ethnology of the Owens Valley Paiute.* University of California Publications in American Archeology and Anthropology, Vol. 33, No. 3.

TALAYESVA, DON C.
1942   *Sun Chief: The Autobiography of a Hopi Indian.* Leo W. Simmons, editor, New Haven: Yale University Press.

TEICHER, M. I.
1960   *Windigo Psychosis: A Study of A Relationship Between Belief and Behavior.* American Ethnological Society Proceedings, Seattle: University of Washington Press.

TEMKIN, OWSEI
1971   *The Falling Sickness: A History of Epilepsy from the Greeks to the Beginnings of Modern Neurology.* 2d ed. Johns Hopkins Press.

TEXTOR, ROBERT B.
1967   *A Cross-Cultural Summary.* New Haven: HRAF Press.

TITIEV, MISCHA
1943   "Notes on Hopi Witchcraft." *Papers of the Michigan Academy of Science, Arts, and Letters* 28:549–37.

1972 *The Hopi Indians of Old Oraibi: Change and Continuity.*
       Ann Arbor: University of Michigan Press.
TYLER, HAMILTON A.
1964 *Pueblo Gods and Myths.* Norman: University of Oklahoma
       Press.
UNDERHILL, RUTH
1948 *Ceremonial Patterns in the Greater Southwest.* American
       Ethnological Society Monograph 13. New York: J. J. Augustin.
VAN WINKLE, NANCY WESTLAKE, AND PHILIP A. MAY
1986 "Native American Suicide in New Mexico, 1957–1979: A
       Comparative Study." *Human Organization* 45:296–309.
VEITH, ELZA
1965 *Hysteria: The History of a Disease.* Chicago: University of
       Chicago Press.
WALLACE, ANTHONY F. C.
1964 *Culture and Personality.* New York: Random House.
WEINSTEIN, EDWIN A.
1962 *Cultural Aspects of Delusion: A Psychiatric Study of the Virgin Islands.* New York: Free Press.
WEINSTEIN, EDWIN A., ROY A. ECK, AND OLGA LYERLY
1969 "Conversion Hysteria in Appalachia." *Psychiatry* 32:334–
       41.
WEST, LOUIS J.
1967 "Dissociative Reaction." In *Comprehensive Textbook of Psychiatry*, edited by Alfred M. Freedman and Harold I. Kaplan,
       885–99. Baltimore: Williams and Wilkins.
WHEELWRIGHT, MARY C.
1951 *Myth of Mountain Chant and Beauty Chant.* Santa Fe: Museum of Navajo Ceremonial Art Bulletin, 5.
WHITE, LESLIE A.
1930 "The Acoma Indians." U.S. Bureau of American Ethnology
       Annual Report 47:17–192.
WHITING, ALFRED F.
1939 *Ethnobotany of the Hopi.* Flagstaff: Museum of Northern Arizona Bulletin, 15.
WHITING, BEATRICE BLYTHE
1950 *Paiute Sorcery.* New York: Viking Fund Publications in Anthropology, 15.
WITHERSPOON, GARY
1977 *Language and Art in the Navajo Universe.* Ann Arbor: The
       University of Michigan Press.

WOOLF,CHARLES M.
1965   "Albinism Among Indians in Arizona and New Mexico."
       American Journal of Human Genetics 17:23–35.
WYMAN, LELAND C.
1936a "Navaho   Diagnosticians."   *American   Anthropologist*
       38:236–46.
1936b "Origin Legends of Navaho Divinatory Rites." *Journal of
       American Folklore* 49:134–42.
1970   *Blessingway.* Tucson: University of Arizona Press.
1975   *The Mountainway of the Navajo.* Tucson: University of Ari-
       zona Press.
WYMAN, LELAND C., AND LORA L. BAILEY
1943   *Navajo Upward Reaching Way: Objective Behavior, Ra-
       tionale, and Sanction.* University of New Mexico An-
       thropological Series Bulletin, 4, #2.
WYMAN, LELAND C., AND CLYDE KLUCKHOHN
1938   *Navaho Classification of their Song Ceremonials.* American
       Anthropological Association Memoir, 10.
YOUNG, ROBERT W., AND WILLIAM MORGAN
1980   *The Navajo Language: A Grammar and Colloquial Diction-
       ary.* Albuquerque: University of New Mexico Press.

Index

Abse, D. Wilfred, 76
Absence seizures (petit mal). See Epileptic seizures
Absentmindedness, 68
Accidents, 35
Agriculture, 24, 28; effects of on tribes, 55, 56, 57, 152–53
Akinesia, 69
Albinism, 70
Alcohol abuse, 10, 42, 44, 45, 81, 99, 100, 129; suicide and, 160, 161. See also individual case histories
Alice (hysteric), case of, 119; hand trembling in, 113–17
Ambivalence, 152, 154, 155, 156–57. See also Gender conflict; Incest; Social isolation of tribes
Amnesia, 119, 120, 126, 137
Anesthesia, 66, 69
Animals, 19, 20, 29, 32
Anna (epileptic), case of: incest and moth madness, 145–47
Annie (epileptic), case of: incest and moth madness, 140–42
Antabuse, 129
Ant doctors, 28
Anthropology: interest of in psychopathologies, 4, 5, 7
Ants, 32
Apache Indians, 8, 10, 18, 31, 32; attitudes toward incest, 16, 52, 56, 58, 153, 167, 168; Chiricahua beliefs and practices, 32, 54, 55, 58; hand-trembling myth, 46; Jicarilla, 55; Lipan, 55; matrilineal descent in, 55, 56; Mescalero, 24, 55, 157; shamans, 102–3
Aphonia, 69
Apollonian traits. See Dionysian/Apollonian personality traits
Appalachia, 76
Arthritis, 94
Asexual children of myth, 50, 52

Athabascan culture, 7, 8, 9, 55
Atonic seizures, 63
Auras, 64, 144
Awonawilona (bisexual god), 49

Badger clan, 25
Bannock Indians, 27
Basso, Keith, 54
Beadway ceremonial, 92
Bears, 32
"Bear" shamans, 27–28
Bear wife, 122
Beauty, concept of, 34
Beautyway ceremonial, 92
Begochidi (bisexual god), 46, 51
Belinda (hysteric), case of, 120–21
Benedict, Ruth, 4–5, 9–10
Betty, case of: incest and moth madness in, 142–43
Bigstarway ceremonial, 91
Bisexual fertility god, 46, 49
Black-Antway-Evil, 91
Blessingway ceremonial, 8–9, 35, 49, 92, 106, 165, 169; importance of, 34–35, 36–37
Blindness, hysterical, 66, 67, 69, 78
Boas, Franz, 21
Body painting, 31
Boyer, L. Bryce, 157, 168
Brain tumors, 61
Breuer, Josef, 68
Brugge, David M., 8
Butterflies: in incest myths, 33, 48, 50, 51, 54. See also White Butterfly (supernatural)
Butterfly People (supernatural), 42, 46, 47, 56

Canyon de Chelly, 56
Carl (epileptic), case of, 122, 131; hand trembling in, 104–7
Carla (hysteric), case of: diagnosis of, 134–35

Cerebrovascular attacks, 61
Ceremonial year, 27
Ceremonies, 1, 2, 12, 20, 34, 169; as
    cause of disease, 32–33. *See also*
    individual ceremonials
Changing Bear Maiden, 90, 91
Chants, 31
Chaos, 29, 97. *See also* Coyote
    (supernatural)
Charcot, Jean Martin, 60, 67, 68, 76
Cheyenne Indians, 152, 160
Childbirth, 5, 34
Child-raising, 155, 157, 158
Children with seizures, 61, 79–80,
    85
Cirrhosis, 143
Clan system, 56. *See also* Endogamy;
    Incest
Clarissa (hysteric), case of, 117, 118,
    119; hand trembling in, 108–9
Cleft palate, 121
Clowns. See *Koyemsi; Paiyatemu*
Comanche Indians, 26, 152–53
Complex partial seizures, 1, 64. *See
    also* Epileptic seizures
Congenital deformities, 121
Consciousness, loss of, 39, 45, 61,
    62. *See also* Epileptic seizures
"Consumption group," 154–55
Contagious magic, 22, 23, 33
Conversion reactions, 68, 69, 114;
    symptoms and disposition of, 76–
    77. *See also* Hysteria;
    Pseudoseizures; *individual reac-
    tions and case histories*
Convulsions, 40, 41, 42, 43. *See also*
    Epileptic Seizures
Coordination disturbances, 69
Corn, 35
Corpse powder, 31, 36
Coyote (supernatural), 9, 15, 24; in
    Apache myth, 53, 150; as cause of
    disease, 122, 130–31, 132; in cere-
    monial myths, 34, 47, 48–49, 94;
    contamination by, 121, 149; in cre-
    ation myths, 29, 159; possession
    by, 23, 31, 46; qualities of, 37, 42,

45, 51, 90, 97; as trickster, 23–24,
    29, 37. *See also* Father-daughter
    incest; Mothway ceremonial
Coyote medicine, 47, 48, 51
Coyote Pass clan, 56
Coyoteway (Luckert), 37
Coyoteway ceremonial, 51, 122, 131,
    169
"Crazy" behavior, 9, 40, 52, 53
Crickets, 32, 33
Crystal gazer, 123
Cultural beliefs: effects of, 4–5, 76–
    77, 168. *See also* Gender conflict;
    Social isolation of tribes
"Culture bound" psychosis, 4
Cuna women, 5
Cyanosis, 63, 144

Dances, 36
Dangerous objects, 32
Datura, 6, 49, 124, 131
Dawn Boy and Dawn Girl, 47
Daydreaming, 68
Deaths of seizure patients, 100, 101,
    141, 143, 144, 145
December (dangerous month), 27
Deer contamination, 123
Depression, 81, 88, 93, 94, 95, 96
Devil, 66
Diagnosis of illness, 2, 5, 30; among
    Navajos, 87–89; problems in, 6–7;
    treatment and, 3–4. *See also* Hand
    trembling; *individual case
    histories*
*Diagnostic and Statistical Manual of
    Mental Disorders*, 69
Diigis, 40–41, 45
Diitła, 40, 43, 44, 103
Dionysian/Apollonian personality
    traits, 9, 10–11, 19, 29–30
Disease, causes of, 9–10, 21, 25–26.
    See also Coyote (supernatural);
    Ghost contamination; Incest; *indi-
    vidual ceremonials and case
    histories*
Diskinesia, 69
Dissociative states, 68, 103, 119, 120

Divination, 2
Division of labor, sexual, 152, 154.
    See also Gender conflict
Divorce, 158
"Doctor" societies, 28
Dreams, 24–25, 44, 94
Dysphoria. See Depression
Dysuria, 140

Eagles, 32
Ego control, Navajo abdication of, 9,
    168
Egypt, 66
Electroencephalograms, 7, 13, 61,
    114, 125, 127, 137
Elizabeth (hysteric), case of, 131;
    frenzy witchcraft and, 123–26
Encephalitis, 61
Endogamy, 54, 58, 70; clan endog-
    amy, 17, 54, 55, 150
Enemy-Monsterway ceremonial, 91,
    121
Enemyway ceremonial, 36, 91, 106
England: surveys from, 71
Epileptic seizures, 1, 40, 136; ancient
    attitudes toward, 3, 60–61; com-
    munity response to epileptics, 80,
    149; complex partial, 64, 98; de-
    scribed, 60–62; epidemiology of,
    70–72, 75; focal (partial), 62, 63–
    65; generalized (grand mal), 16–
    17, 40, 62–63, 64; "Jacksonian"
    seizures, 64; Navajo treatment of,
    97–98; petit mal (absence), 63;
    psychomotor (complex partial), 1,
    64; simple partial, 64; symptoms,
    42–43, 60–65. See also individual
    case histories and ceremonials
Eskimos, 152
Evil, concept of, 34
Evil spirits: as cause of disease, 32.
    See also Ghost contamination
Evilway ceremonials, 36, 49, 91, 146;
    blackening ritual, 114, 121, 135;
    reddening ritual, 135; Upward-
    reachingway, 96, 97; uses of,
    93–94

Excreta (hair, nails, feces) in spells,
    31
Exogamous clans, 55, 56, 57
Extreme behavior, 41–42, 45

Fainting spells, 33, 44
Falret, Jules, 66
False pregnancy, 69
Family structure: Navajo, 154–58
Father: conflict with, 130–32. See
    also individual case histories
Father-daughter incest, 16, 17, 54,
    151; concern about, 150, 161–62,
    165–67; Coyote myths and, 165–
    67; reasons for attitudes toward,
    56, 57, 58, 59
Febrile seizures, 61
February (land purified), 27
Fertility ceremonies, 24
Fire, 29
Fire ceremony, 47
First Man, 31
Flintway ceremonial, 46, 91
"Flower Mound," 51
Focal seizures (partial). See Epileptic
    seizures
Fort Defiance, 11, 12
Frazer, James, Sir, 21
Frenzy witchcraft, 6, 17, 41, 119;
    father-daughter incest and, 166–
    67; uses of, 1, 2, 32, 54, 55. See
    also individual case histories
Frenzy-witchcraftway ceremonial,
    131, 169; medicines in, 51; myths
    about, 48–49, 50, 150; occasions
    performed, 91, 98, 110, 112, 122,
    127, 128
Freud, Sigmund, 4, 68–69
Friedrich, Nikolaus, 66
Fright, sudden, 20, 40, 53
Fugue states, 98, 104, 105, 126, 133
Funerals, 79

Galen, 66
Gambling, 2, 32, 41
Gameway ceremonial, 122, 131;
    smoking ritual, 123

Gender conflict, 29, 37; pastoralism and, 152, 157, 158–61
Generalized seizures. *See* Epileptic seizures
Ghost contamination, 22, 33, 36, 40, 94; as cause of disease, 33, 106; changing times and, 168–69; examples, 114, 128, 134, 135
Gila Monster (supernatural), 2, 30, 41, 46
Globus hystericus, 116, 117
Good/bad thoughts: power of, 25–26, 29–30, 52, 97
Goodwin, Grenville, 58
Gossip, 155, 156
Gough, Kathleen, 57
Grand mal (generalized) seizures. *See* Epileptic seizures
Grasshoppers, 32, 33
Greece, ancient: beliefs about seizures, 60, 65, 66
Gutman, David, 12, 111, 115, 130, 135, 146

Haemophilus influenza, 75
Hail storm, 32
Haile, Berard, 47, 48
Hallucinations, 1, 77, 106
Hand trembling, 5–6, 15, 41; epileptics and, 104–7; as gift, 30–31; hand tremblers as shamans, 102–3; hysterics and, 107, 117–18; signs of, 102–4. *See also individual case histories*
Hand-tremblingway ceremonial: myths about, 31, 46; occasions performed, 91, 108, 109, 116
Hauser, W. Allen, 71
Head trauma, 61, 62
Healers, Hopi, 25, 26, 122, 126, 127
Hegar, Alfred, 66
Henderson, Eric B., 169
Hermaphrodite children of myth, 49, 52
"Highway hypnosis," 68
Hippocrates, 66

Hiram, case of: father-daughter incest, 162–65
Hoebel, E. Adamson, 152
Holy People (supernatural), 32, 35
Holyway ceremonials, 35, 36
Homicide, 10, 81; patterns of, 158, 160
Hopelessness, feelings of, 94, 95
Hopi Indians, 8, 15, 48; attitude toward incest, 150–51; attitude toward shamans, 37–38; development of society of, 24–27; disposition of seizure cases among, 70–72, 73–74, 75, 78, 79; incest myths, 51, 52; suicide among, 161. *See also* Pueblo Indians
Hunter/gatherer societies, 19, 20, 24, 28–29
Hunting, 2, 32, 143; hunt god, 29; rituals, 36, 51, 54; supernatural beliefs about, 19, 20
Hyperventilation, 66, 81
Hypnosis, 67, 68
Hypoxia, 61
Hysteria, 2, 3, 4; described, 65–69; epidemiology of, 75–79; moth madness and, 133–34; Navajo treatment of, 97–98; symptoms, 9, 10, 76. *See also individual case histories and ceremonials*
"Hysterical overlay," 77, 81
"Hystero-epilepsy," 67

Iceland: surveys from, 71, 76
"Idiopathic" epilepsy, 61
Illegitimate children, 99, 129, 141
Imitative magic, 22
Inanimate forms, 20
Incest, 6; Apache myths, 53–55; clan incest, 52, 56; Mothway for, 47–48; Navajo descriptions of, 45–46; Pueblo myths, 49–53; purposes of beliefs, 55–59; punishment for, 51, 52, 53–54, 152–53; reasons for concern, 150–51; tribes compared, 152–53. *See also* Father-daughter

incest; Moth madness; Sibling incest; Social isolation of tribes
Incontinence, 63, 90, 126, 142, 144
India, 76
Indian Health Service, 14, 71
Individual: importance of, 23, 25–26, 37; Pueblo ideal of, 29–30
Infantile spasms, 63
Inflammatory disease, 72, 75
Interviews and case histories, 13; love magic, 52–53; patients' self-descriptions, 43–46. See also individual case histories
Isolation of families. See Social isolation of tribes

Jackson, Hughlings, 60
"Jacksonian" (simple partial) seizures. See Epileptic seizures
Japan: shamans in, 102
Jealousy, 160, 161
Jemez Indians, 8
Johnson, Dale, 9

Kahun medical papyrus, 65
Kaplan, Bert, 9, 168
Kaska Indians, 153
Katcinas, 27, 35
Keresan, 8, 27–28, 29, 49. See also Pueblo Indians
Kluckhohn, Clyde, 54, 154, 155
Korea: shamans in, 102, 103
Koshare, 50
Koyemsi (clowns), 49, 50–51
Kretschmer, Ernst, 67
Kroeber, Alfred, 102, 103
Kunitz, Stephen J., 88, 93
Kurland, Leonard T., 71
Kwakiutl shaman, 21

Laura (epileptic), case of, 121–22, 144–45
Lévi-Strauss, Claude, 5, 21
Levy, Jerrold E., 88, 93, 108, 134, 146
Life and death in ceremonial year, 27
Lifeway ceremonial, 35, 36, 91, 121, 145

Lightning, 25, 34; as cause of disease, 28, 32, 33, 122
Listeners, 30, 46
Llewellyn, Karl N., 152
Love magic, 52, 53, 54, 55, 59, 131, 166. See also Frenzy witchcraft
Lowie, Robert H., 157
Luckert, Karl, 9, 37

Madmen, 26
Marriage: disapproved marriages, 161; marital discord in myth, 159–60. See also Gender conflict
Mary (epileptic), case of, 130, 131; frenzy witchcraft and, 126–30; hand trembling and, 107
Masau (god of death), 27
Masked dancers, 35
Masks, 31
Matrilineal societies, 8, 54, 150, 158; effects of on tribes, 56, 57, 58
Medication, antiepileptic, 72, 78, 85, 123, 129, 139, 141, 144
Medicinal plants, 51
Men: disposition of seizure cases among, 81–84; hysteria in, 78–79, 99; role of in family, 158–61. See also Ambivalence; Gender conflict
Meningitis, 61, 75
Mental illness: Navajo attitudes toward, 94, 95–97
Mental retardation, 40, 45, 63, 80, 104
Metrazol potentiation, 140
Mildred (hysteric), case of, 117, 119, 122, 131–32; hand trembling in, 109–13
Mimicry, 67
Mono tribe, 27
Monsters, mythical, 33
Moth madness, 1; described, 41; signs of, 133. See also Incest; individual case histories
Moth medicine, 47, 48, 51
Moths, 32, 33, 34
Mothway ceremonial, 1, 42, 51, 169;

Mothway ceremonial, *continued*
account of, 47–48; Coyote rituals
as substitute for, 90, 91, 133; as
extinct, 89–90; myths about, 34,
42, 46–47, 56, 150; relation to incest beliefs, 56, 57–58
Mountain soil bundle, 35
Mountaintopway (or Mountainway)
ceremonial, 51, 90–91, 94, 143,
169; smoking ritual, 122, 123, 127
Moving-upway ceremonial. *See* Upward-reachingway ceremonial
Muingwu (fertility god), 51
Murphy, Jane, 102
Music, 50
Myoclonic seizures, 63
Myths, 5, 34, 36–37, 159–60; creation myths, 19–20, 28–29, 31, 37.
See also Coyote (supernatural); *in-
dividual ceremonials*

Natural phenomena as cause of disease, 32
Navajo Indians, 1, 75; adaptations
from Pueblo contact, 30–36; attitudes toward shamans, 37–38;
community reaction to incest and
seizures, 79–81, 85–86; disposition of seizure cases among, 70–
71, 72, 73–74, 77, 78; history and
religion, 7–9, 10, 11, 15, 169. *See
also* Epileptic seizures; Hysteria;
Puebloization; *individual case histories and ceremonials*
Negamide potentiation, 137
Neurophysiology, 68
Neurosis, 4
Neutra, Raymond, 14
Newekwe clowns, 50
Nightway ceremonial, 35, 47, 91
"Non-sunlight-struck maidens,"
172n.3
Numic speakers, 27

Obsession, 45
Oedipal conflict, 68, 69, 130
Ojibwa, 4

Okinawa: shamans in, 102
Orpheus myths, 22
Ovariectomies, 66

Paiute Indians, 24, 26
Paiyatemu (trickster), 49, 50
Paralysis, hysterical, 66, 69, 78, 104,
126
Paraphernalia, ceremonial, 25, 34, 35
Parasthesia, 69
Parker, Dennis, 14, 43, 107, 108, 115
Partial dissociative reactions, 68
Partial seizures secondarily gener-
alized, 64. *See also* Epileptic
seizures
Pastoralism, 17, 151–52, 157–58; ef-
fects of, 167–68
Patrilineal descent, 157–58
"Patterns of Culture" (Benedict), 4
Petit mal seizure. *See* Epileptic
seizures
Peyote, 103, 104
Phratries, 54, 172n.5
Plains tribes, 20
Plumeway ceremonial, 92
Pollen, 35
Polygynous marriages, 162
Porcupines, 32
Possession, 26, 34, 37, 41, 103, 168
Postencephalopathy, 72
Postictal twilight state, 63, 129
Poverty and epilepsy, 70–71
Prayer ceremony, 135
Priests, 20, 27
Prodrome, 64
Promiscuity, 99. *See also* Coyote (su-
pernatural); Sexual excess;
individual case histories
Pseudoseizures, 2, 3, 5–6, 81; de-
scribed, 65–69; epidemiology of,
75–79
Psychological problems, 65, 79–81
Psychomotor seizures (complex par-
tial). *See* Epileptic seizures
Psychopathologies, 4; culture and, 6–7.
See also Hysteria; Pseudoseizures
"Psychophysiologic disorder," 76

Psychosocial environment, 68, 69, 98, 99
"Psychosomatic medicine," 76
Psychotherapy, 3–4
Psychotic behavior, 1, 4, 65, 81. See also individual case histories
Puberty ritual, 34
Pueblo Indians, 8; attitudes toward incest, 15, 52, 55, 56–57; community attitude toward seizures, 40, 70, 85–86; influence of, 24–30, 35; personality traits of, 10, 11, 19; social controls among, 155–56. See also Incest; Navajo
Puebloization, 8, 17, 151
Pueblo Revolt of 1680, 8, 56
Purification ceremonies, 27, 79

Rabid Coyote, 90, 145
Rabid dog contamination, 127, 128, 174n.3
Radin, Paul, 24
Rain ceremonies, 24, 28
Randomness and chance, 23–24
Rape, 99, 149
Rattles, 36
Raven, 23–24
Research methods, 11–15, 71–72, 88–89, 93
Riverward Knoll, 46, 51
Robert (epileptic), case of, 143–44
Rome, 66

Sand paintings, 31, 105, 107, 142, 146
Schizophrenia, 5, 45, 111
Seizures: defined, 60–62; discrimination of type, 97–101; patients' self-description of, 39–42. See also Epileptic seizures; Hysteria; Pseudoseizures
Separation of sexes, 59
Sexual conflict. See Gender conflict
Sexual deviation, 37, 59
Sexual excess, 59, 90, 159–60. See also Coyote (supernatural)

Shamans, 5, 15, 102–3; in North American tribes, 19–24; powers of, 26, 27–28, 37–38
Shaman societies, 28, 171n.4
Shock, 33
Shootingway ceremonial, 34, 91, 121, 122, 123, 135, 145, 146
Shoshone Indians, 20–21, 24, 26
Siberia: shamans in, 103
Sibling incest, 2, 13, 31, 50, 52, 150; association with seizures, 15–16, 17; epileptics and, 147–49; reasons for attitudes toward, 55, 56–57, 151. See also Moth madness; individual case histories and tribes
Simple partial seizures, 64. See also Epileptic seizures
Singers, 30, 108, 109, 117, 169
Sings. See individual ceremonials
Snake doctors, 28
Snakes, 32
Snapping Vagina, 91. See also Vagina dentata.
Social controls of behavior, 151, 154, 155, 156, 164
Social isolation of tribes, 58, 70; fear of incest and, 151, 153–57, 161, 166
Social stigmatization, 6, 17
Somatization, 76, 95, 115
Son of Old Man Hat, 159–60
Sorcery, 31, 54
Soul loss, 9, 22–23, 25, 26, 33, 37, 168
Spells, 31
Spirit helpers, 22
Stargazers, 30, 31, 34, 46, 109
Status epilepticus, 63
Stevenson, Matilda Cox, 52, 53
Sucking cure, 15, 21, 22, 122, 126
Suckingway ceremonial, 32, 110, 111
Suicide, 10, 70, 79, 97, 121, 126; attempts, 81, 129, 144; patterns of, 158, 160–61
Summer: ceremonies in, 36
Summer solstice, 27
Sun, 46, 50

Supernatural beliefs of North American tribes, 19–24
Surveys on seizures, 71, 75, 76
Susan (epileptic), case of, 122, 131; frenzy witchcraft and, 123
Sympathetic magic, 21
Symptoms. *See individual types of seizures*

Tabus, breach of, 21, 23, 25, 31; emphasis on, 26–27, 35; by parents, 41, 46; during pregnancy, 32–33. *See also* Father-daughter incest; Incest; Sibling incest
Takic languages, 27
Tanoan shamans, 27–28
Temporal lobe epilepsy, 136
Tetany, 144
Tewa Indians, 8, 14–15, 28, 51, 52; disposition of seizure cases among, 71, 72, 73–74
Thematic Apperception Test, 12, 111, 125, 130, 135, 146, 147
Thunderbird doctors, 28
Titiev, Mischa, 26
Tonic-clonic (*grand mal*) seizure. *See* Epileptic seizures
Trading, 32
Trance states, 5, 20–21, 25, 31
Transvestite, 142
Treatment of illness, 4, 5. *See also* Sucking cure; *individual ceremonials*
Trickster figures, 23–24, 29. *See also* Coyote (supernatural)
"Trotting Coyote," 166
Tuba City, 11, 12–14
Tunnel vision, 69
Turning Basket ritual, 91, 106, 108, 122, 123
Twins, 25

U.S. Public Health Service, 7
Upward-reachingway ceremonial, 36, 96–97

Ute, 8, 26, 32
Uto-Aztecan language, 27

Vagina dentata, 29, 174n.2
Violence. *See* Alcohol abuse; Homicide; Psychosis
Vision quest, 20, 24
Vomiting, 69
Vows, 25

War ceremonies, 36
Water, 32
Weather forecasting, 29
Were-animals, 44, 54, 155
Whirling Coyote ritual, 90, 128, 174n.3
Whirlwinds, 32, 33
White Butterfly (supernatural), 48, 51
Wilfred (epileptic), case of: incest and moth madness in, 136–40
Wind, "evil," 34, 51, 52
Wind concept, 33
Windigo, 4
Windway ceremonial, 34, 91, 122, 145, 146; Chiricahua, 107, 121
Winter: ceremonies in, 36
Winter solstice, 27
Witchcraft, 6, 21, 31, 94, 121
Witches, 22, 25, 53, 54; powers of, 31, 26–27
"Witches sabbath," 54
"Witch father-in-law" theme, 166
Wizardry, 32, 54, 110
Women, 76; disposition of seizure cases among, 6, 78, 81–84; illnesses of, 65, 66–67, 69; status of, 157–58. *See also* Ambivalence; Gender conflict
Wyman, Leland C., 36

Zuni Indians, 8, 14; attitudes toward incest, 151; attitudes toward shamans, 27–28; disposition of seizure cases among, 70–72, 73–74, 75, 78, 79; incest myths, 49, 50–52. *See also* Pueblo Indians

About the Authors

Jerrold E. Levy, professor of anthropology at the University of Arizona since 1972, received his Ph.D. in 1959 from the University of Chicago. The focus of his academic interest has been the study of Indian health problems. With Stephen J. Kunitz, Levy co-authored *Indian Drinking: Navajo Practices and Anglo-American Theories* (John Wiley & Sons, 1979).

Raymond Neutra, Chief of Epidemiological Studies and Surveillance Section, California Department of Health Services, received his M.D. from McGill in 1965 and his Dr.P.H. from Harvard in 1974. He has taught both at Harvard and at the University of California, Los Angeles.

Dennis Parker (1912–1984) was a Navajo Indian, born and raised on the reservation. Tuberculosis kept him in sanatoria in Arizona and California for fifteen years; there he learned to read and write Navajo and he translated two books of the New Testament. Parker attributed his survival to modern medicine and dedicated the rest of his life to promoting the better health of his people, working as a medical interpreter, as an aide in Community Health Education, and as a mental health technician. After retirement, he continued to collaborate with Levy until his death.